THE ESSENTIAL EBUS BRONCHOSCOPIST©

rake press

Laguna Beach, CA

THE ESSENTIAL EBUS BRONCHOSCOPIST

BRONCHOSCOPY INTERNATIONAL™

Murgu S and Colt HG Second Edition 2015

THE ESSENTIAL EBUS BRONCHOSCOPIST©

The Essential EBUS Bronchoscopist© is the second volume of the Essential Bronchoscopist™, a series of books containing numerous question/answer sets pertaining to the art, science, techniques and overall practice of bronchoscopy. This series attempts to cover major elements of cognitive, affective and experiential knowledge, and technical skill needed to become a competent bronchoscopist. Each volume of the series also serves as a major reading assignment of the Bronchoscopy Education Project, an officially endorsed endeavor striving to create a uniform approach to the teaching, training, and practice of bronchoscopy around the world.

The Essential EBUS Bronchoscopist© is comprised of a single module, containing a specific competency-oriented list of learning objectives and thirty multiple choice question sets. These are also viewable on line in several languages (www.Bronchoscopy.org and www.essential-bronchoscopy.org). Information pertains to major topics related to endobronchial ultrasound and EBUS-guided transbronchial needle aspiration, including ultrasound physics, mediastinal anatomy, patient preparation, indications contraindications and complications, bronchoscopic technique, image acquisition, radiographic interpretation and ultrasound image pattern recognition, equipment malfunction and troubleshooting, nodal sampling strategies, specimen collection, and expected results for diagnosing and staging lung cancer and other disorders involving the mediastinum. This module pertains only to convex-probe EBUS and does not cover in detail radial-probe based interventions.

The aim of The Essential EBUS Bronchoscopist© is to enhance the learner's progress along the learning curve from novice to competent practitioner. To encourage interactive learning and communication among peers, many question/answer sets are intentionally written so that a correct response is not readily apparent. Sometimes, as in real life, more than one answer may be acceptable to the learner. Other times, the learner or their mentors may disagree with what is written. We hope these differences of opinion and practice will enrich the reader's experience, and serve as a helpful addition to their affective and experiential knowledge base.

At the end of the module is a set of ten post-test questions that should ideally be answered after reading the module. Questions may also be used during didactic lectures or as part of pretest-posttest sessions at regional meetings conducted as part of Bronchoscopy International inspired training sessions. None of these questions are meant to serve as high stakes tests, but rather as low-stakes continuing self-learning assessments that help document the progressive acquisition of knowledge needed for the safe and competent practice of EBUS and EBUS-guided TBNA.

Henri G. Colt MD, FCCP

The Essential Bronchoscopist™ Series includes

- The Essential Flexible Bronchoscopist©
- The Essential EBUS Bronchoscopist©
- The Essential Intensivist Bronchoscopist©
- The Essential Interventional Bronchoscopist©
- The Essentials of Bronchoscopy Education©

rake
press

Bronchoscopy International, Laguna Beach, CA 92651

Murgu Septimiu and Colt Henri G
The Essential EBUS Bronchoscopist© Second Edition, 2015
From, The Essential Bronchoscopist™ series

ISBN 978-0-9848347-3-0

1. The Essential Flexible Bronchoscopist©
2. The Essential EBUS Bronchoscopist©
3. The Essential Intensivist Bronchoscopist©
4. The Essential Interventional Bronchoscopist©
5. The Essentials of Bronchoscopy Education©

Manufactured in the United States of America

1 2 3 4 5 6 7 8 9 10

THE ESSENTIAL EBUS BRONCHOSCOPIST

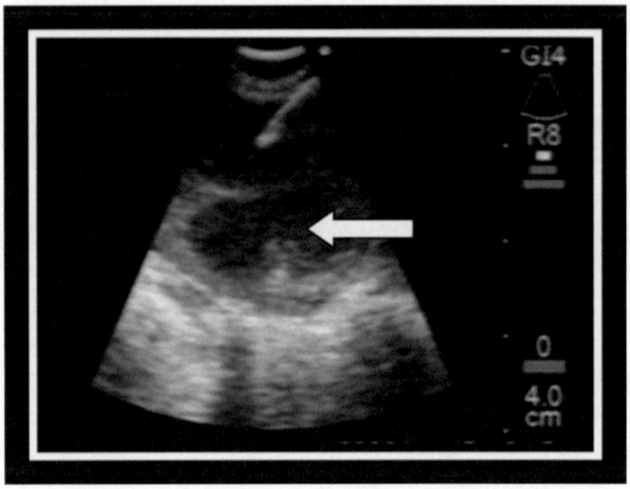

Exploring the Mediastinum with Endobronchial Ultrasound and EBUS-TBNA

Funding statement

Funding for The Essential EBUS Bronchoscopist© is a result of Dr. Colt's philanthropic endeavors and from the general support of the University of California, Irvine. No corporate support was either solicited or received for this work.

EBUS Bronchoscopist© Disclaimer

Confidentiality of data potentially relating to individual patients and visitors has been respected. We strive to honor or exceed any legal requirements of medical/health information privacy as they apply to the United States and to the state of California.

Images and case descriptions provided here-in, therefore, are not intended for the diagnosis of any specific patient. Any information found on the website or in this text should not be used as a substitute for medical care.

The authors disclaim liability, injury, or damage incurred as a consequence from the use of information. Reference to websites, instruments, or equipment portrayed in this material is not of commercial nature, nor does the inclusion imply endorsement.

Should documents or images from this material be copied for personal use, we request that materials remain unedited and unmodified unless for teaching purposes, that no fee be charged for copies or access to the information, that copyright notices and disclaimers remain attached, and that credit be given to The Essential EBUS Bronchoscopist© (suggested format Essential EBUS Bronchoscopist© www.bronchoscopy.org

The Essential EBUS Bronchoscopist

Learning bronchoscopy in the world today

"Learning Endobronchial Ultrasound and EBUS-TBNA -related theory"

TABLE OF CONTENTS

§

THE EBUS BRONCHOSCOPIST©

The EBUS Bronchoscopist© has been intentionally designed for adult self-guided learning of endobronchial ultrasound (EBUS) and endobronchial ultrasound-guided transbronchial needle aspiration (EBUS-TBNA) related theory. This reading material is best used to complement educational programs that provide patient-based learning experiences and participation in postgraduate continued medical education programs with incorporated hands-on instruction using simulation-based scenarios. The major focus of this text is convex-probe EBUS, therefore, very little information pertaining to the techniques of radial-probe EBUS is provided.

In order to provide a uniform approach to learning EBUS-related theory, The Essential EBUS Bronchoscopist© contains thirty modular question-answer sets, which, can be used in conjunction with posters, assessment tools, patient-centered practical approach exercises and instructional videos in order to assist learners become competent EBUS bronchoscopists. The enlightened EBUS Bronchoscopist will gradually develop an individual approach to this exciting procedure. Practice, a curiosity to question conventional wisdom, and a desire for self-improvement will ultimately lead to improved technical skill that will enhance patient care around the globe. It is our hope, however, that the materials included in this text and in the companion Endobronchial Ultrasound and EBUS-guided TBNA Training Manual will help accelerate the learner's progress along the procedural learning curve, and help assure greater uniformity and structure to the procedural education process.

We would like to thank our friends and colleagues Dr. Pyng Lee from the National University Hospital, Singapore, Dr. Mohsen Davoudi, from the University of California, Irvine, and Dr. David Fielding from the Royal Brisbane Hospital, Brisbane, Australia for their advice in bringing this work to fruition.

We expect to modify and expand on this text in the years ahead, and very much look forward to your input and suggestions on how to make this text more inclusive and of even greater value to learners. Please do not hesitate to contact us at www.Bronchoscopy.org with questions, comments, ideas and suggestions.

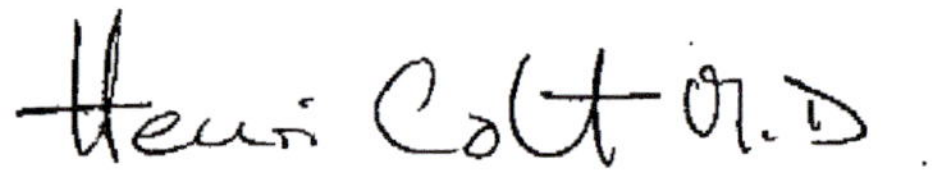

Henri Colt MD., FCCP

MODULE I

THIRTY MULTIPLE CHOICE QUESTION/ANSWER SETS

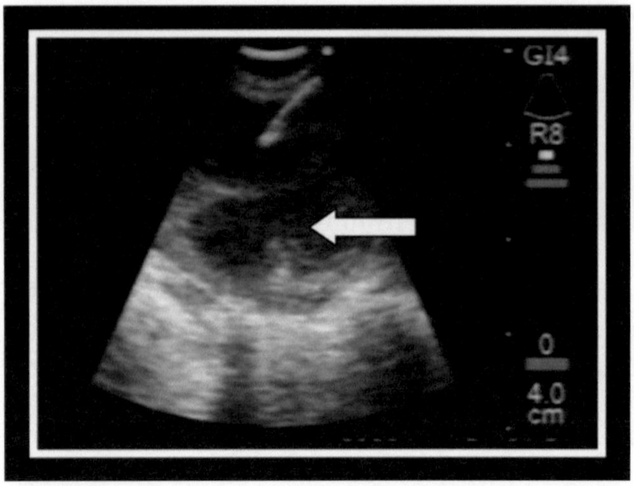

LEARNING OBJECTIVES

Readers of **The Essential EBUS Bronchoscopist©** should not consider this a test. In order to most benefit from the information contained here-in, every response should be read regardless of your answer to the question. You may find that not every question has only one "correct" answer. This should not be viewed as a trick, but rather, as a way to help *you* think about a certain problem. Expect to devote approximately 2 hours of continuous study completing the 30 question-answer sets.

A multiple choice 10 question post-test addresses specific elements of the learning objectives The Essential EBUS Bronchoscopist©. Questions may at times, be related to other learning materials contained in instructional videos, posters, or slideshows relating to EBUS and EBUS-TBNA. While a 70% correct response is often considered a satisfactory grade, we recommend that you target a score of 100%.

At the conclusion of this Module, the learner should be able to:

1. Describe at least four artifacts seen during EBUS and EBUS-TBNA.
2. Describe the various differences between high and low frequency ultrasound.
3. Describe situations in which EBUS-TBNA might be associated with or replaced by EUS-FNA or other methods of mediastinal exploration.
4. Identify at least three measures that help improve quality ultrasound image acquisition.
5. Describe how inadvertent wrist movements might alter the ultrasound image and how this might affect patient safety.
6. Describe techniques of EBUS-TBNA and recognized elements of an adequate, representative cytology sample.
7. Describe at least 3 different strategies that help obtain a diagnostic sample.
8. Describe nodal sampling strategies in various cases of known or suspected malignant pulmonary lesions that help assure accurate staging.
9. Describe the roles for EBUS radial probe and convex probe various malignant and benign lung, airway, and mediastinal disorders.
10. Describe EBUS-TBNA related indications, techniques, complications, and expected outcomes using evidence from the literature.

§

User Instructions

Recommended reading of
The Essential EBUS Bronchoscopist© with post-tests

The *Essential EBUS Bronchoscopist©* is a laddered curriculum of theoretic bronchoscopic knowledge. It has been prepared with the assistance and input of several EBUS experts worldwide who contributed question/answer series or advice. This and other materials can be downloaded from The Bronchoscopy International website (www.Bronchoscopy.org) an HON code certified (Health on the Net) voted by the American Thoracic Society as the best on-line resource for bronchoscopy education, and officially endorsed by numerous professional medical organizations worldwide. This reading assignment is complementary to other learning materials contained in the Endobronchial Ultrasound and EBUS-TBNA program of the respected Bronchoscopy Education Project officially endorsed by the World Association for Bronchology and Interventional Pulmonology (WABIP).

The aim of the *Essential EBUS Bronchoscopist* © is to complement a traditional apprenticeship model of training in EBUS and EBUS-TBNA by emphasizing important facets of knowledge and skill required for competency. Elements addressed in the *Essential EBUS Bronchoscopist* © are intentionally written so that contrary opinions might occasionally be provided by instructors. In this fashion, dialogue is promoted, but access to a certain amount of "essential" material is guaranteed. The question-answer sets of the *Essential EBUS Bronchoscopist©* contain information pertaining to mediastinal and hilar nodal and vascular anatomy, lymph node mapping, scope insertion and placement within the airways, patient preparation, indications, contraindications and complications, techniques and solutions to technical problems, image processing and troubleshooting, ultrasound physics and image artifacts, site specific pattern recognition, as well as lung cancer staging and restaging. This question answer set is also available as an interactive PowerPoint presentation.

In order to document that a learner has been exposed to material contained in the *Essential EBUS Bronchoscopist* ©, a passing score of 70 and above (7/10 correct responses) is recommended to consider the module completed on the EBUS Bronchoscopy Education Competency Checklist (see EBUS checklists and assessment tools manual at www.Bronchoscopy.org).

Question I.1: A 71 year old Chinese woman presented to the outpatient clinic with weight loss and a chronic cough of 3 months' duration. Her medical history included hypertension and hemithyroidectomy 20 years ago for Graves' disease. Chest radiograph revealed a left paratracheal mass with contralateral tracheal deviation. A chest computed tomography scan revealed retrosternal goiter with an enlarged left lower paratracheal lymph node. Bronchoscopy with conventional TBNA of the left lower paratracheal lymph node obtained blood and was nondiagnostic. A possible next step is to:

A. Perform thyroid function tests for this likely benign disorder
B. Proceed with open mediastinal exploration.
C. Proceed with EBUS-TBNA of the left lower paratracheal lymph node.
D. Proceed with CT guided transthoracic needle aspiration of the thyroid mass.

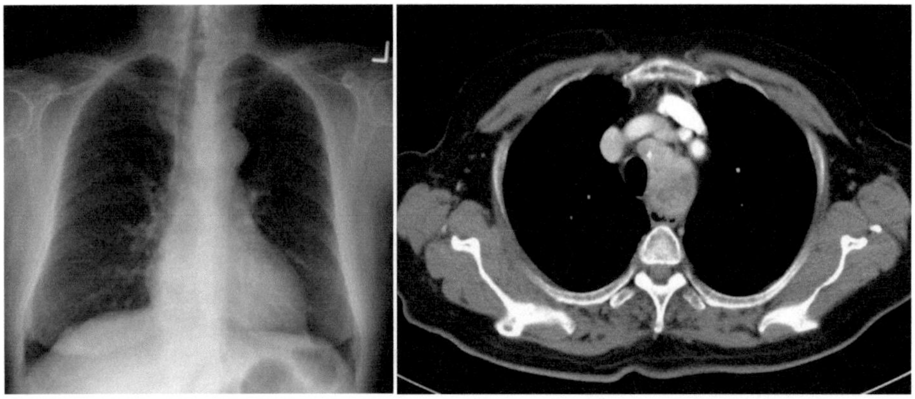

Answer I.1: C.

Mediastinal goitres represent about 10% of mediastinal masses[1]. Computed tomography findings include encapsulation, lobulation, heterogeneity, and continuity between cervical and mediastinal components. While thyroid function tests should be performed, histologic diagnosis is warranted because malignancy develops in a number of mediastinal goiters

EBUS-guided TBNA represents an alternative to percutaneous needle aspiration or open surgical exploration[2, 3]. Proposed indications for EBUS-TBNA include negative conventional TBNA, staging the radiologically normal mediastinum in suspected or confirmed lung cancer, mediastinal restaging after induction chemotherapy, and diagnosis of mediastinal, hilar, peribronchial, paratracheal, or intrapulmonary masses[4]. In this case, needle aspiration of the lymph node as well as of the retrosternal goiter revealed clusters of follicular cells consistent with benign thyroid tissue

REFERENCES:

1. Duwe BV, Sterman DH and Musani AI. Tumors of the mediastinum. Chest 2005;128;2893-909.
2. Steinfort DP, Irving LB. Endobronchial Ultrasound Staging of Thyroid Lesion in Small Cell Lung Carcinoma Thorac cardiovasc Surg 2010;58: 128-129.
3. Chalhoub M, Harris K. The use of endobronchial ultrasonography with transbronchial needle aspiration to sample a solitary substernal thyroid nodule. Chest 2010;137:1435-6.
4. Yasufuku K, Nakajima T, Chiyo M, Sekine Y, Shibuya K, Fujisawa T. Endobronchial ultrasonography: current status and future directions. J Thorac Oncol 2007;2:970-9.

Question I.2: A patient with a history of cough, fatigue and PET avid mediastinal and hilar lymphadenopathy is referred for EBUS-TBNA. The lower right paratracheal lymph node is shown below. Which of the following sonographic characteristics is the most specific for a metastatic lymph node?

A. Its heterogeneous echogenicity

B. Its short axis of 1.5 cm

C. The hypoechoic areas within the lymph node without blood flow

D. Its distinct margins

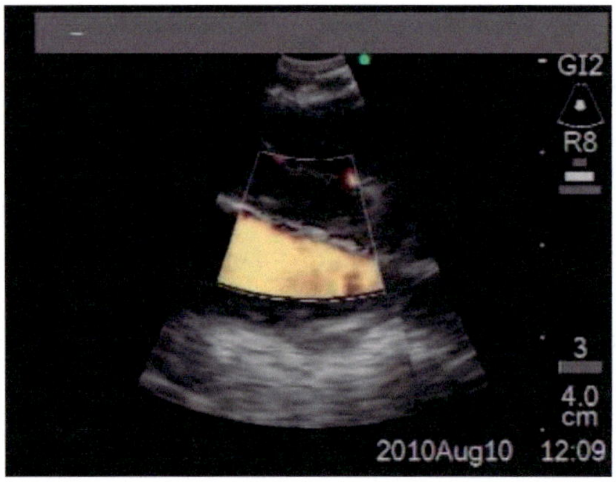

Answer I.2: C

The node in question is greater than 1 cm in short axis, has round shape, is heterogeneous, has distinct margins, has a central necrosis sign (CNS) and lacks central hilar structure (CHS). Sonographic features are useful in the evaluation of lymph node metastasis in head and neck cancers, breast cancers and thoracic malignancies[1, 2]. A large study evaluating 1061 lymph node stations from 487 patients with confirmed or suspected lung cancer reported the utility of morphologic sonographic features of mediastinal and hilar lymph nodes using

EBUS in order to predict presence or absence of metastasis[3]. The lymph nodes were characterized based on EBUS imaging as follows:

a) Size (in short axis): less or more than 1 cm

b) Shape: oval or round; when the ratio of short vs. long axis of lymph nodes is smaller than 1.5, the lymph node is defined as round; if the ratio is bigger than 1.5, it is oval.

c) Margin: indistinct or distinct; if the majority of the margin (>50%) is clearly visualized with a high echoic border, the lymph nodes are determined as distinct. If the margin is unclear, they are determined as indistinct.

d) Echogenecity: homogeneous or heterogeneous

e) The presence or absence of central hilar structure (CHS); CHS defined as a linear, flat, hyperechoic area in the center of the lymph node.

f) The presence or absence of coagulation necrosis sign (CNS). CNS is a hypoechoic area within the lymph node without blood flow. Typical coagulation necrosis sign represents a low echoic area within the lymph node and that sometimes occupy the majority of the lymph node.

EBUS characteristic	**Sensitivity**	**Specificity**	**PPV**	**NPV**	**Diagnostic accuracy**
Heterogeneous echogenicity	77.3%	86.6%	69.5%	90.6%	83.9%
The size greater than 1 cm	77.9 %	75.8%	55.9%	89.7 %	76.4%
The presence of CNS	69.4%,	92.6%,	78.9%,	88.4%	86.0%
The presence of distinct margins	94.4%	54.3%	45.5%	96.0%	65.7%

The presence of CNS had the highest specificity (92.6%) and the highest hazard ratio (5.6) for prediction of metastatic lymph nodes. These data do not obviate the need for sampling the node but the high negative predictive values could be useful. For instance, if a bronchoscopist performs EBUS-TBNA on a lymph node in a patient with suspected lung cancer and the cytological specimen is adequate and reveals only benign lymphocytes, then this is the instance when the lack of the lymph node EBUS malignant characteristics can be reassuring in confirming its true negativity.

REFERENCES:

1. Lee N, Inoue K, Yamamoto R, et al. Patterns of internal echoes in lymph nodes in the diagnosis of lung cancer metastasis. World J Surg. 1992;16: 986-94.
2. Bhutani MS, Hawes RH, Hoffman BJ. A comparison of the accuracy of echo features during endoscopic ultrasound (EUS) and EUS-guided fine-needle aspiration for diagnosis of malignant lymph node invasion. Gastrointest Endosc. 1997; 45:474-9
3. Fujiwara T, Yasufuku K, Nakajima T et al. The utility of sonographic features during endobronchial ultrasound-guided transbronchial needle aspiration for lymph node staging in patients with lung cancer: a standard endobronchial ultrasound image classification system. Chest. 2010;138:641-7.

Question I.3: While performing EBUS-TBNA, you notice that the lymph node being sampled moves but that the needle does not enter it. What should be done next?

A. Abort the procedure
B. Change to a conventional bronchoscope with larger histology needle
C. Change the puncture site
D. Proceed with aspiration anyway

Answer I.3: C

There is usually no reason to abort the procedure or switch to a conventional bronchoscope. Often the needle does not penetrate the node because of the thick capsule of the node, or because the needle is hitting airway cartilage. In the Figure below, images A, B and C were captured at three consecutive moments during EBUS-TBNA. Please notice the LN (the isoechoic oval structure) and its capsule (the hyperechoic line) moving away from the transducer, suggesting that the needle has not penetrated the capsule. In most cases, retracting the needle into the scope, and slightly changing the position of the EBUS scope while still maintaining view of the lymph node, will allow penetration of the node when the needle is advanced again more forcefully, while sometimes minimally changing the position of the needle hub (sheath) on the airway wall. Aspiration should not be performed unless the lymph node is obviously penetrated, as the aspirate will likely reveal benign bronchial cells and be nondiagnostic.

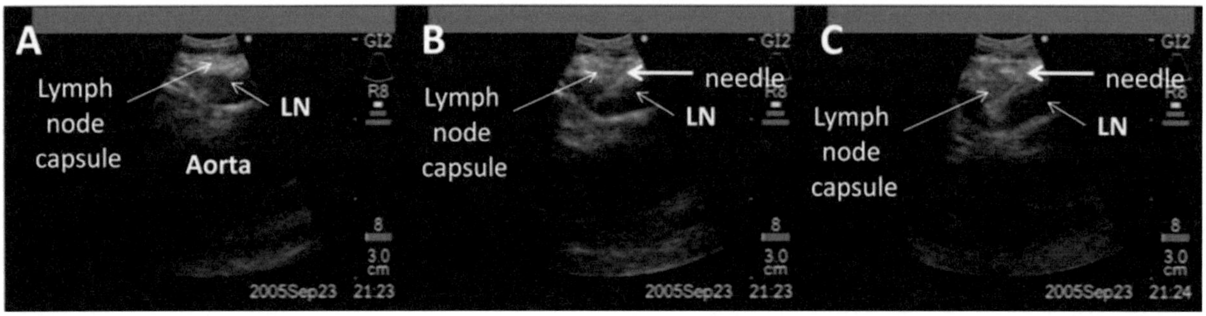

Question I.4: While performing EBUS-TBNA from a subcarinal lymph node (level 7), you obtain a bloody aspirate. This is because:

A. The inferior pulmonary vein has been penetrated.

B. The left atrium has been penetrated.

C. The right pulmonary artery has been penetrated

D. A blood vessel within the lymph node itself has been penetrated

Answer I.4: D.

Each of the anatomic structures listed; inferior pulmonary vein, left atrium, and right pulmonary artery could be inadvertently penetrated during EBUS-TBNA of a level 7 node. However, this would suggest that the node itself is not being visualized during needle insertion, or that the scanning plane is more anterior rather than medial (as it should be for visualizing this station). Blood vessels inside a lymph node are not uncommon and can be visualized as hypoechoic structures that are Doppler positive.

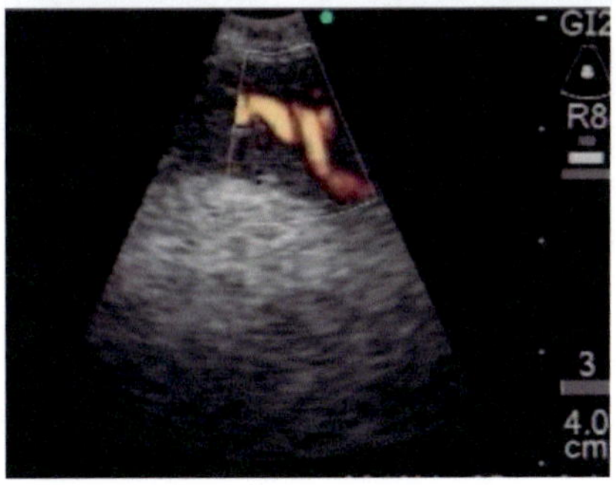

Question I.5: While performing EBUS-TBNA, you have just completed aspiration while watching the needle deep within a lymph node (image A). You are now interrupted by your assistant asking whether she should call for your next patient. You then notice image B on your display screen. What happened?

A. You accidently retracted the needle

B. You inadvertently changed your wrist position while holding the scope and changed the scanning plane of the EBUS-bronchoscope.

C. You assistant changed the penetration depth on the image processor without telling you.

D. You assistant pulled the needle and sheath out without telling you.

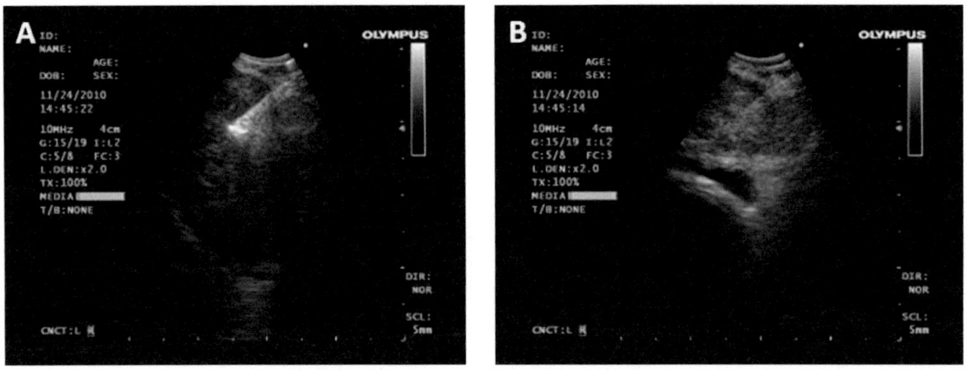

Answer I.5: B.

It is unlikely that you accidently retracted the needle because you should be watching each and every movement of the needle while you are aspirating the lymph node. You should also be watching the needle as you retract it back into its sheath and give the command to unlock the needle-sheath device in order to remove it. It is also unlikely that your assistant pulled the needle and sheath out without telling you, because the needle-sheath ensemble is locked into place on the working channel of the EBUS scope. The penetration depth on the image processor has not been changed because the same distance measurements (right hand side of the images) are visible on both image A and B. It is likely that in turning your head to speak with your assistant, you also rotated your wrist in such a way that you changed the scanning plane of the ultrasound while the needle remained in the same position. Note that the images displayed are different, consistent with different scanning planes. While this does not affect diagnostic yield, it may result in accidental puncture of structures adjacent to the node because the tip of the needle is not visualized. It is possible that distractions of any sort during operative procedures can adversely impact patient safety.

REFERENCES

1. Weigmann DA, ElBardissi AW, Dearani JA et al. Disruptions in surgical flow and their relationship to surgical errors: an exploratory investigation. Surgery 2007;142:658-665.

Question I.6: For a patient with a 3.2 x2.5 cm right upper lobe mass confirmed as adenocarcinoma by CT guided FNA, and a 1.1 cm right lower paratracheal lymph node seen on computed tomography, the best diagnostic yield for staging prior to thoracotomy is offered by:

A. Esophageal ultrasound-guided fine needle aspiration (EUS) alone

B. Endobronchial ultrasound –guided transbronchial needle aspiration (EBUS) alone

C. Mediastinoscopy

D. Combined EUS and EBUS followed by Mediastinoscopy

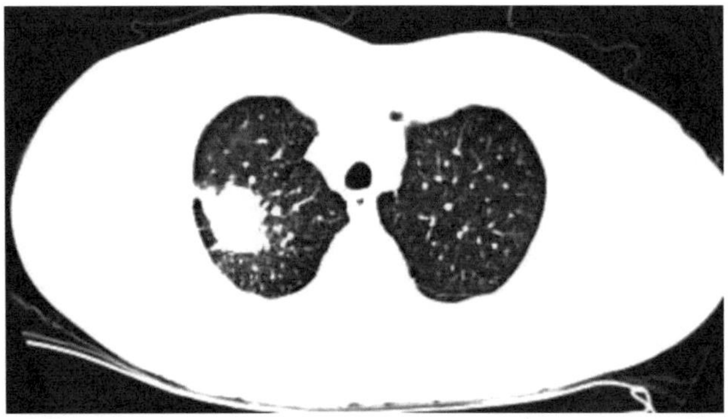

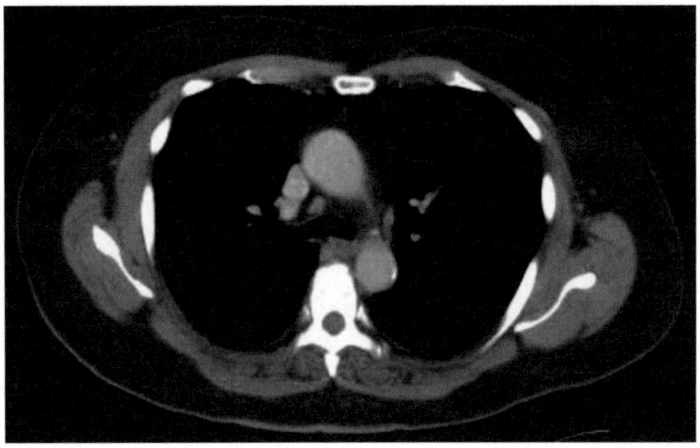

Answer I.6: D.

Clinical staging of lung cancer is an integral part of patient care because it directs therapy and has prognostic value. In cases of resectable primary tumor and absence of distal metastasis, mediastinal nodal involvement directs treatment, with surgical resection of the tumor being the treatment of choice in the absence of mediastinal nodal metastases[1], whereas combined modality treatment is indicated for patients with mediastinal nodal metastases[2]. EUS alone is suitable for assessing lymph nodes in the posterior aspect of lymph node stations 4L, 5 and 7 and in the inferior mediastinum at stations 8 and 9. EUS alone has limited value for complete staging because right-sided nodes are usually inaccessible. Mediastinoscopy provides systematic exploration and biopsy under visual guidance of nodal stations 1, 2, 3, 4 and 7. EBUS alone provides no access to lymph node stations 5, 6, 8 and 9. A staging strategy combining endosonography (EUS and EBUS) and mediastinoscopy (if no nodal metastasis were detected at endosonography) resulted in greater sensitivity for mediastinal nodal metastases and fewer unnecessary thoracotomies (needed in only 1 of 7 patients) in comparison with mediastinoscopy alone[3] when thoracotomy was used as the reference standard.

REFERENCES:

1. Scott WJ, Howington J, Feigenberg S, Movsas B, Pisters K; American College of Chest Physicians. Treatment of non-small cell lung cancer stage I and stage II: ACCP evidence-based clinical practice guidelines (2nd edition). Chest. 2007;132(3)(suppl):234S- 242S.
2. Robinson LA, Ruckdeschel JC, WagnerH Jr, Stevens CW; American College of Chest Physicians. Treatment of non-small cell lung cancer-stage IIIA: ACCP evidence-based clinical practice guidelines (2nd edition). Chest. 2007;132(3)(suppl):243S- 265S.
3. Annema JT, van Meerbeeck JP, Rintoul RC et al. Mediastinoscopy versus ednosonography for mediastinal nodal staging of lung cancer: a randomized trial. JAMA. 2010;304:2245-2252

Question I.7: A 69 year old patient with 30 pack-year history of smoking was found to have a 2 cm left upper lobe nodule and mediastinal lymphadenopathy. EBUS-TBNA from the right (4R) and left (4L) lower paratracheal lymph nodes showed reactive lymphocytes but no malignancy. The next step is to:

A. Proceed with EUS to repeat biopsy from station 4L.

B. Perform mediastinoscopy.

C. Proceed with thoracotomy with nodal dissection.

D. Refer to oncology for multimodality treatment for stage III B lung cancer.

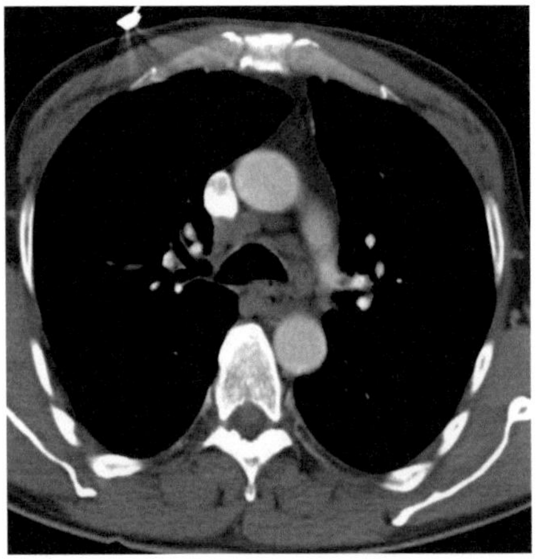

Answer I.7: B.

Indeed EUS provides access to station 4L, but the yield of diagnosis at this level is similar to that of EBUS[1]. EUS does not provide access to station 4R, which, if positive in this patient will upstage the tumor to III B. Thoracotomy with nodal dissection in this patient with highly suspected mediastinal nodal disease is neither cost effective nor necessarily therapeutically advantageous. While stage III B is likely in this patient with contralateral lymphadenopathy, tissue confirmation is necessary because computed tomography or PET are known to be of low sensitivity for staging. In one study, up to 28% of patients with a high clinical suspicion of nodal disease had mediastinal nodal metastases confirmed by mediastinoscopy despite negative EBUS-TBNA[2]. Therefore, a negative EBUS-TBNA in patients with highly suspected mediastinal nodal involvement based on CT or PET should be followed by mediastinoscopy.

REFERENCES:

1. Herth FJ et al. Am J Respir Crit Care Med 2005; 171: 1164-1167
2. Defranchi SA, Edell ES, Daniels C E et al. Mediastinoscopy in Patients With Lung Cancer and Negative Endobronchial Ultrasound Guided Needle Aspiration. Ann Thorac Surg 2010; 90: 1753– 8

Question I.8: A 42 year old nonsmoking woman was diagnosed with a 4 cm lung mass and bulky (2 cm in short diameter) bilateral mediastinal lymphadenopathy (station 4R, 4L, 7) suggesting at least stage III B lung cancer. The oncologist asks you to obtain diagnosis and provide enough specimens for molecular analysis. In order to achieve this you should:

A. Ask your surgical colleagues to perform a mediastinoscopy to obtain a large surgical specimen from the lymph nodes.
B. Proceed with EBUS-TBNA to obtain the at cytology specimens for molecular analysis.
C. Tell the oncologist that there is no role for such testing.
D. Ask your interventional radiology colleagues to perform a CT –guided biopsy from the lung mass.

Answer I.8: B.

Low volume cytology specimens such as those obtained via EBUS-TBNA are adequate for molecular analysis such as EGFR and ALK[1, 2]. Furthermore, EBUS-TBNA would provide diagnosis and staging in one setting. Therefore, mediastinoscopy is not warranted if a less invasive procedure could achieve the same goal. A CT-guided FNA will also provide cytology and possibly a core histology specimen; this procedure, however, would only make the diagnosis of the lung mass, and contrary to EBUS-TBNA, does not provide mediastinal staging. Studies support the benefits of targeted therapy in NSCLC. Molecular analysis is becoming standard practice for advanced NSCLC. As of this writing, however, tests are mostly warranted in patients with adenocarcinoma and minimal or no smoking history.

REFERENCES

1. Garcia-Olive´ I, Monso´ E, Andreo F, et al. Endobronchial ultrasound-guided transbronchial needle aspiration for identifying EGFR mutations. Eur Respir J. 2010;35: 391-395.
2. Sakairi Y, Nakajima T, Yasufuku K et al. EML4-ALK Fusion Gene Assessment Using Metastatic Lymph Node Samples Obtained by Endobronchial Ultrasound-Guided Transbronchial Needle Aspiration. Clin Cancer Res; 16(20); 4938–45.

Question I.9: While performing EBUS-TBNA, you notice the following image on the display monitor. What has happened?

A. You rotated your wrist and now you are imaging a blood vessel..

B. The lymph node is not in the scanning plane and you are imaging the normal lung

C. The balloon is not in intimate contact with the airway wall.

D. Nothing has happened; this is the normal pattern of a lymph node.

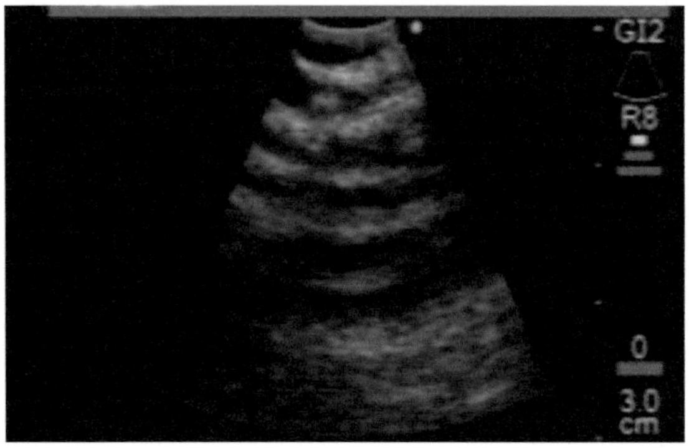

Answer I.9: C.

Fluid (blood) transmits the ultrasound completely so that blood vessels have the least echogenicity during EBUS, therefore, they often appear black (anechoic) (Figure A). The normal lung being filled with air, on the other hand, is hyperechogenic and appears white (Figure B). The lymph nodes are usually well defined structures with isoechoic (comparable with the surrounding tissue) or mixed hypoechoic, isoechoic, or hyperechoic pattern, depending on their content (Figure C). The pattern in the question is characterized by multiple equally spaced strong hyperechoic lines on the ultrasound image, due to acoustic waves being repeatedly reflected between the airway wall and the transducer. This is called reverberation artifact and occurs when the balloon of the EBUS scope is not in contact with the airway wall (Figure D).

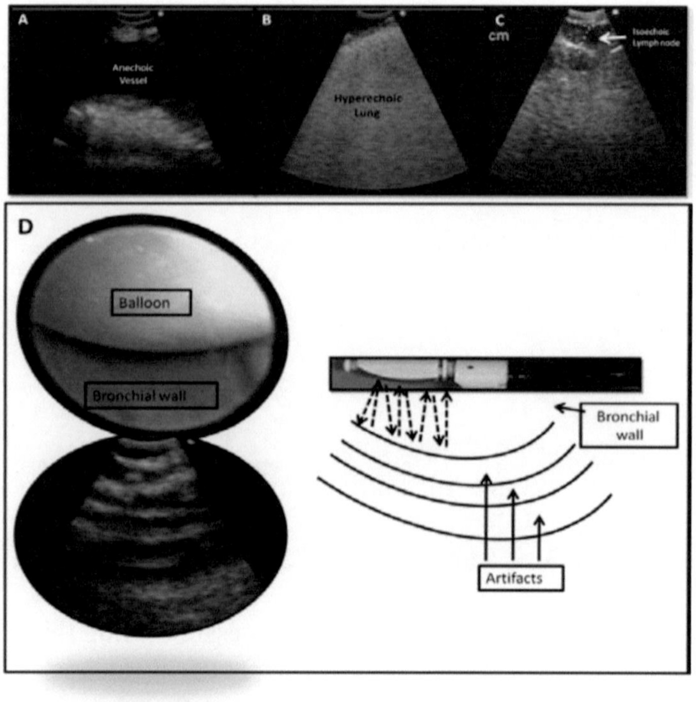

Question I.10: Which of the following lymph node stations can be sampled by EBUS-TBNA?

A. Station 5 (subaortic; aorto-pulmonary window).

B. Station 6 (para-aortic).

C. Station 7 (subcarinal).

D. Station 8 (paraesophageal).

E. Station 9 (pulmonary ligament).

Answer I.10: C.

EBUS-TBNA offers access to all stations adjacent to the trachea or bronchi (2, 4, 7, 10, 11) (Figure). However, level 5, 6, 8 and 9 lymph node stations, while sometimes visualized via EBUS, by not being adjacent to the airway, are not accessible using this technique. Station 5 and 6 can be approached by through an anterior mediastinotomy), while stations 8 and 9 can be approached via EUS-FNA or thoracoscopy.

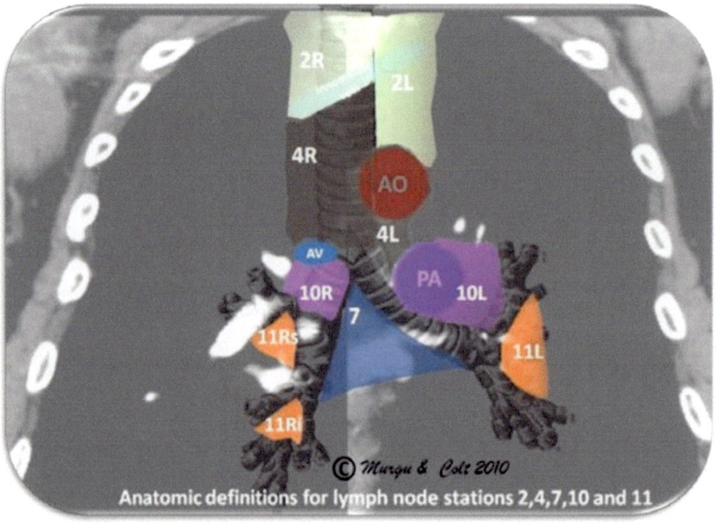

Anatomic definitions for lymph node stations 2,4,7,10 and 11

Question I.11: During an EBUS-TBNA staging procedure in a patient with a left upper lobe mass and lymphadenopathy at level 10L, 7, 4L and 4R, you initially start by sampling which of the following nodes?

A. Station 10L

B. Station 7

C. Station 4L

D. Station 4R

Answer I.11:D.

For this patient with a left upper lobe mass, station 10L is an ipsilateral N1 node, and stations 7 and 4L are N2, while station 4R is a contra lateral mediastinal node (N3). Complete sonographic mediastinal and hilar nodal assessment is necessary during EBUS-TBNA for staging purposes because the tumor may be upstaged to N3 (Stage III B), in case EBUS identifies contra lateral lymph nodes from which aspirates are positive for malignancy[1]. EBUS-TBNA is performed first from N3 nodes, followed by N2 nodes, and if needed for diagnostic purposes N1 nodes. If N3 nodes were found to be positive for malignancy on rapid on-site cytological evaluation, the procedure could be terminated. At this time, from a staging perspective, determining N1 positivity does not alter therapeutic strategies. No benefit has been shown for providing neoadjuvant chemotherapy to patients with known N1 disease, and patients with N1 lymph node involvement are not denied resection if they have an acceptable risk profile for surgery[2]

REFERENCES:

1. Herth F, Lunn W, Eberhardt R, et al. Transbronchial versus transesophageal ultrasound guided needle aspiratin of enlarged mediastinal lymph nodes. Eur Respir J 2006; 28: 910-914
2. Shrager J. Mediastinoscopy: Still the Gold Standard. Ann Thorac Surg 2010;89:S2084 –9

Question I.12: After two aspirates from the subcarinal lymph node in a patient with suspected lung cancer, the cytologist tells you that the Diff-Quick stain shows scant lymphocytes and benign bronchial cells. You should:

A. Continue the procedure and perform another one or two aspirates.
B. Abort the procedure and wait for the final results.
C. Abort the procedure since the specimen shows lymphocytes.
D. Continue the procedure until a diagnosis is obtained.

Answer I.12: A.

An EBUS-TBNA cytology specimen is considered adequate or representative if there is presence of frankly malignant cells, granulomas or lymphocytes, lymphoid tissue, or clusters of anthracotic pigment-laden macrophages[1]. Higher yields may be obtained by obtaining aspirates from the periphery of the node. Therefore, the procedure should be continued and another one or two aspirates should be performed with the intent to sample other regions of the lymph node. Aborting the procedure because lymphocytes are seen and assuming the specimen is representative is premature. The specimen is considered inadequate or non-representative if there are no cellular components, scant lymphocytes (defined as <40 per HPF), blood only, cartilage or bronchial epithelial cells only[2]. A quantitative cut-off value of at least 30% cellularity composed of lymphocytes has been arbitrarily proposed by some experts[3]. There is a good correlation between rapid on-site evaluation and the final cytologic diagnosis, so aborting the procedure hoping that the final result will be diagnostic is not an appropriate next step. However, during

EBUS-TBNA, the diagnostic yield plateaus after a mean of three aspirates. Optimal results can be obtained in three aspirations per lymph node station. When at least one tissue-core specimen is obtained by the first or second aspiration, two aspirations per station can be acceptable. Therefore, continuing the procedure “indefinitely” thinking that eventually a diagnosis will be made is also not warranted and may increase the risk for complications from prolonged sedation, anesthesia, or procedure related complications such as pneumothorax, bleeding, bacteremia, pericarditis, mediastinitis, or scope breakage.

REFERENCES:

1. Alsharif M, Andrade RS, Groth SS et al. Endobronchial ultrasound-guided transbronchial fine needle aspiration : the University of Minnesota experience, with emphasis on usefulness, adequacy assessment, and diagnostic difficulties. Am J Clin Pathol 2008; 130 (3): 434-443.
2. Lee HS, Lee GK, Lee HS et al. Real-time endobronchial ultrasound guided transbronchial needle aspiration in mediastinal staging of nonsmall cell lung cancer : how many aspirations per target lymph node station. Chest 2008; 134(2): 368-374.
3. Trisolini R, Lazzari A, Patelli. Conventional vs endobronchial ultrasound-guided transbronchial needle aspiration of the mediastinum. Chest 2004; 126(3): 1005-1006.

Question I.13: This EBUS image is obtained while imaging the left lower paratracheal lymph node station. Which of the four structures labeled A, B, C or D represents the aorta?

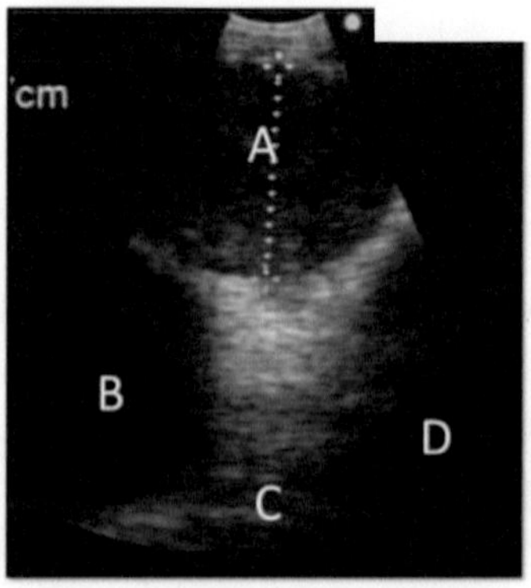

Answer I.13: D.

The upper border of lymph node (LN) station 4L (left lower paratracheal) is the superior margin of the aortic arch (Ao) and the lower border, the upper rim of the left main pulmonary artery (PA). This LN is located lateral to the trachea at the level of main carina. In order to visualize it using EBUS, the scope should be in the lower trachea the level of main carina. The transducer is turned towards the left to visualize the paratracheal region[1]. The coronal computed tomography view identifies the EBUS scanning plane and reveals the same structures but in different positions (see Figure below). To understand the EBUS image based on the CT scan, however, several reference points must be understood

- The EBUS image is projected on the monitor as if the scope is horizontal.
- The green dot on the monitor represents the point where the needle exits the scope and corresponds to the superior (cephalad) aspect of the body.

- This dot is by default towards the 1'o'clock (orientation based on patient being scoped from the head) position of the screen.

If one rotates the CT image clockwise in order to horizontalize the scope and bring the green dot cephalad towards the 1 o'clock position, the two images (CT and EBUS) correlate and show all structures in the same locations. Because the green dot corresponds to the more cephalad, and therefore proximal aspect of the body, the vascular structure at approximately 3 o'clock (D) is the Aorta (proximal), while the vascular structure at 9 o'clock (orientation based on patient being scoped from the head) (B) is the pulmonary artery (distal). The LN (A) is adjacent to the airway in between the two vessels, while the hyperechogenic density in between the Ao and PA is the lung parenchyma at the level of the AP window (C).

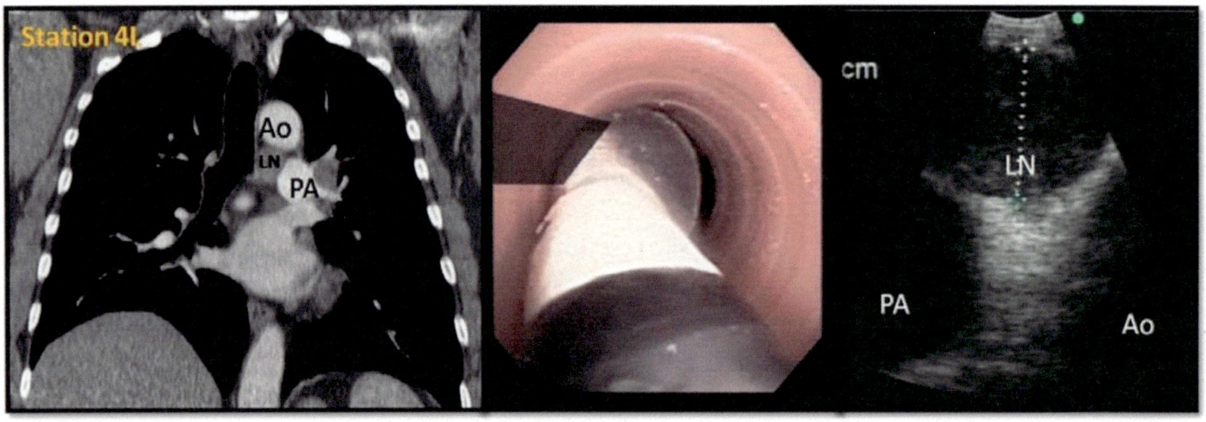

REFERENCES:

1. Murgu S and Colt HG. Practical approach to planning endobronchial ultrasound-guided transbronchial needle aspiration of left lower paratracheal lymph node (level 4L). Egyptian J Bronch 2009;3(2):169-171.
2. Murgu S and Colt HG. EBUS-CT-Bronchoscopy correlations poster and digital media learning aid (posted 2010). http://www.youtube.com/watch?v=3ccrA6hSRqA. Available on You Tube (BronchOrg site).

Question I.14: With the EBUS scope placed just proximal to the main carina and turned towards the 3-o'clock position (orientation based on patient being scoped from the head), the following EBUS image is displayed. The visualized lymph node represents:

A. Station 4R

B. Station 10R

C. Station 2R

D. Station 7

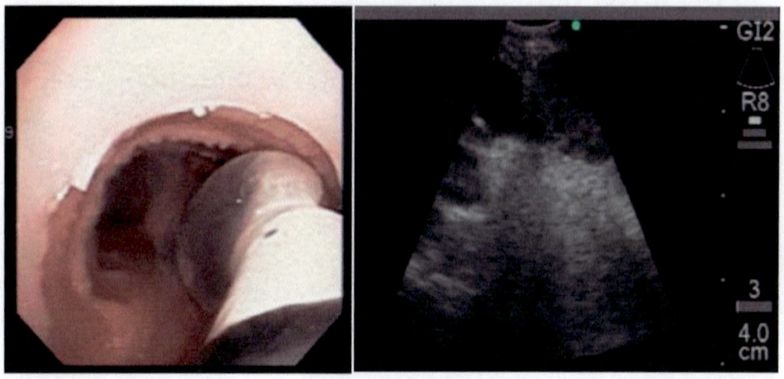

Answer I.14: A.

At this location, with the scope scanning laterally towards the right lateral wall of the trachea, the anechoic round structure at 11o' position on the EBUS image represents the azygous vein (orientation based on patient being scoped from the head). The isoechoic structure seen above it at 1 o'clock position (orientation based on patient being scoped from the head) represents the right lower paratracheal lymph node (4R). Station 4R includes right lower paratracheal nodes, and pretracheal nodes extending to the left lateral border of trachea. The upper border is the intersection of the caudal margin of the innominate vein with the trachea while the lower border is the lower border of azygos vein. Station 2R includes nodes extending to the left lateral border of the trachea. The upper border is the apex of the right lung and pleural space, and in the midline, the upper border of the manubrium while the lower border is the intersection of caudal margin of the innominate vein (IV) with the trachea. Station 10R includes nodes immediately adjacent to the right main bronchus and hilar vessels including the proximal portions of the pulmonary veins and main pulmonary artery. The upper border is the lower rim of the azygos vein and the lower border is the interlobar region between the RUL and Bronchus Intermedius. Station 7 is the subcarinal nodal station with the upper border comprised of the carina of the trachea and the lower border comprised by the upper border of the lower lobe bronchus on the left and the lower border of the bronchus intermedius on the right.

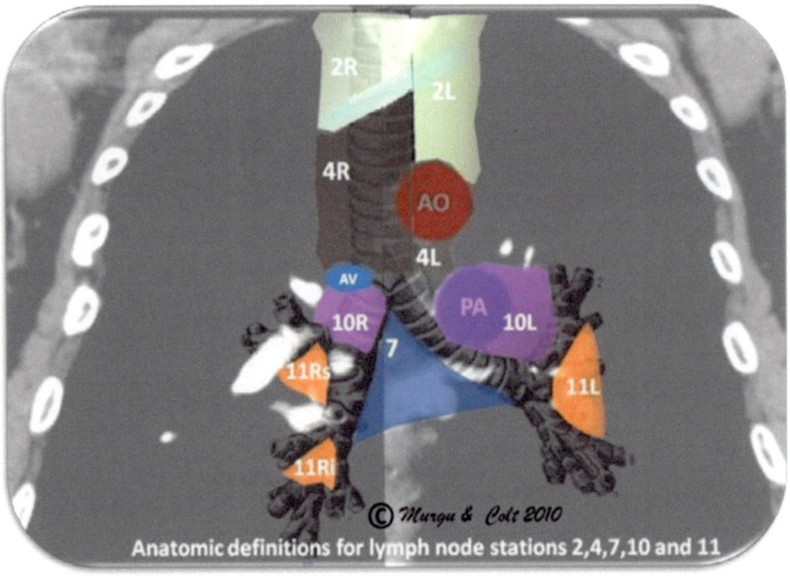

Question I.15: A patient is referred for EBUS-TBNA from the subcarinal lymph node. The CT scan is shown below. Your EBUS scope is out for repair and expected to be returned in several days. The patient and his referring doctor would like to proceed with a diagnostic intervention as soon as possible. What is the most appropriate next step?

A. Wait until the EBUS scope is available and then proceed with EBUS-TBNA
B. Refer the patient to your gastroenterologist colleague for EUS-FNA
C. Refer the patient to your thoracic surgery colleague for mediastinoscopy
D. Proceed with conventional TBNA with rapid on-site examination

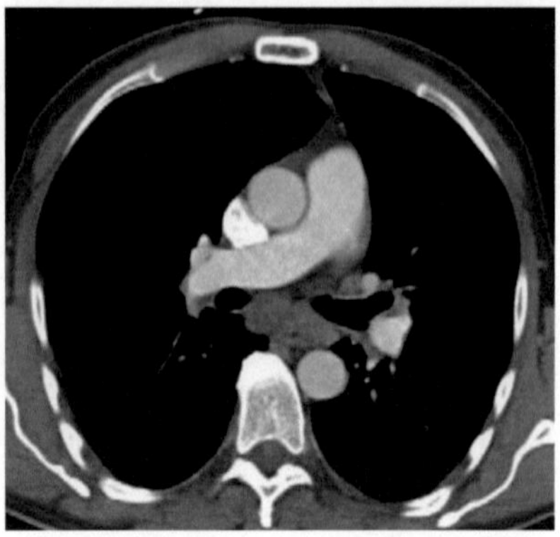

Answer I.15: D.

One could argue that waiting for the EBUS scope is appropriate. If diagnosed with lung cancer, this would be a stage IIIA (with bulky lymphadenopathy) and the patient will likely initiate multimodality treatment rather than undergo primary surgical resection. Delaying diagnosis for several days will not impact management. Both the patient and the referring physician, however, wish to obtain a diagnosis as soon as possible. EUS-FNA and mediastinoscopy have a high diagnostic yield for subcarinal lymph nodes, but might delay the diagnosis because necessary specialist consultations may not always be readily available; furthermore, mediastinoscopy is more invasive and with higher complication rates than needle aspiration techniques (if one excludes possible false-negative EBUS-TBNA as a complication). Conventional TBNA with rapid on site examination is an appropriate next step in this patient if diagnosis is rapidly desired. This patient has no other lymph nodes visible on computed tomography. The yield of conventional TBNA for large subcarinal lymph nodes is similar to that of EBUS-TBNA. In all other cases (except 4R in some studies), EBUS guidance significantly increases the yield compared with conventional TBNA[1].

REFERENCES:

1. Herth F, Becker H, and Ernst A. Conventional versus ultrasound-guided transbronchial needle aspiration: a randomized trial. Chest 2004; 125:322–325.

Question I.16: While performing EBUS-TBNA you notice the hyperechoic structure distal to the node in the figure shown below (see arrows). This represents:

A. Air bronchogram.

B. Tadpole tail sign.

C. Acoustic shadow artifact.

D. Comet tail artifact.

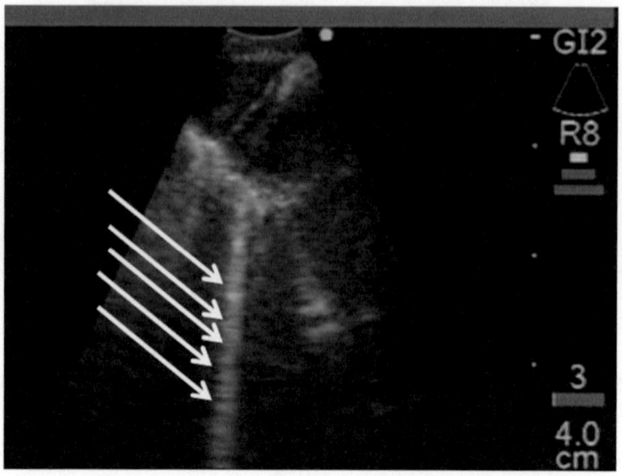

Answer I.16: B.

The hyperechoic structure distal to the node represents the tadpole tail sign, a form of attenuation artifact. Attenuation artifacts include the tadpole tail sign and the acoustic shadow artifact. Tissues with low acoustic impedance such as necrotic lymph nodes, mediastinal cysts and blood vessels result in lower attenuation than tissues with higher impedance[1]. The tadpole tail artifact occurs when the echo at the distal border of the low impedance structure is higher, in which case ultrasound displays the area distal to the low impedance structure more brightly compared to the surrounding tissue. In this case, the low impedance structure is represented by the short linear hypoechoic structure representing a blood vessel inside the lymph node (see Figure below).

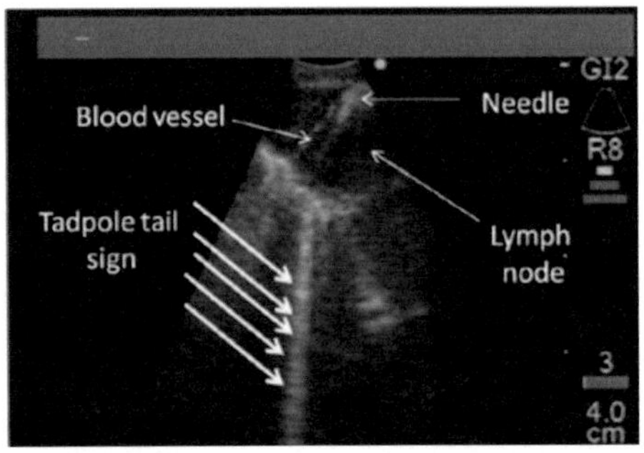

The acoustic shadow artifact is the exact reverse of the tadpole tail. The area behind a high impedance structure is displayed with lower brightness than the rest of the surrounding tissue. Because the ultrasound beam is almost completely reflected at the border or attenuated within the high impedance structure, the area behind it appears as a hypoechoic dark shadow. Comet tail artifacts are a subtype of reverberation artifacts. In tissues containing two highly reflective surfaces (air bubbles, calcifications), this reverberation artifact can be seen if the structures are very small and the two reflective borders are close to each other, in which case the reverberation artifact appears distally to the structure like a comet tail[1]. Air bronchograms present sonographically as hyperechoic foci within a consolidated lung, suggesting that the bronchus supplying the affected area is still patent. This photograph does not reveal a consolidated lung, which sonographically has the same echogenicity as the liver, hence the term sonographic "hepatization" of the lung.

REFERENCES:

1. Nishina K, Hirooka K, Wiegand J, Dremel H. Principles and Practice of endoscopic ultrasound. In Boliger CT et al (eds): Clinical Chest Ultrasound: From the ICU to the bronchoscopy suite. Prog Respir Res. Basel, Karger, 2009, vol 37,pp 110-127.
2. Murgu S, Saffari, A, Davoudi M, and Colt HG. Physics of endobronchial ultrasound. http://www.youtube.com/watch?v=5cxwBjOlF-M&feature=related. You Tube, posted October, 2010.

Question I.17: While imaging the left lower paratracheal region in a Doppler mode you notice this image shown below on the display monitor. The anechoic Doppler negative structure in the right lower corner on the display monitor represents:

A. A mediastinal cyst

B. Necrotic mass

C. Aorta

D. Pleural effusion

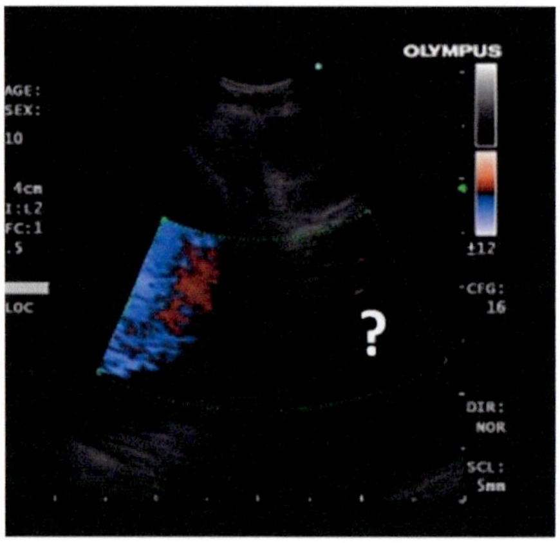

Answer I.17: C.

This image represents a characteristic pattern of the left lower paratracheal lymph node (station 4L)[1]. The structure at the 12 c'clock position is the lymph node, the Doppler positive structure is the pulmonary artery while the anechoic structure, even though Doppler negative in this case, is the aorta. Doppler Effect (shift) represents the phenomenon through which the frequency of the reflected US wave is changed when it strikes a moving object, such as red blood cells within blood vessels. Color Doppler (Duplex Scanning) refers to a color code used to indicate flow direction and velocity. The Doppler Effect is described by the following equation: Doppler frequency shift= $\Delta F = Ft - Fr = 2 \times Ft \times (v/c) \times \cos\theta$, where Ft=transmitted frequency, Fr=received frequency, v=speed of moving target, c=speed of sound in soft tissue, θ=angle between the direction of blood flow and direction of the transmitted sound phase. In general, the Doppler angle (θ) needs to be 60 degrees or slightly less to the long axis of the vessel to obtain the correct velocity. If the angle is 90 degrees, then the $\Delta F = Ft - Fr = 2 \times Ft \times (v/c) \times \cos 90 = 0$, thus resulting in no frequency shift and no "Doppler signal". If the ultrasound scanning plane is perpendicular to the direction of blood flow within a vessel, it is possible that there will be no Doppler signal[2]. This should not lead to misinterpretation of the vessel as a non-vascular structure, such as in this case. In fact, by gently twisting the wrist, the Doppler angle will change and a Doppler signal will be obtained, consistent with a vascular structure (see Figure below). All other processes in the question may present with anechoic Doppler negative pattern, but since they are not vascular structures, they will remain Doppler negative after changing the scanning plane position and the Doppler angle.

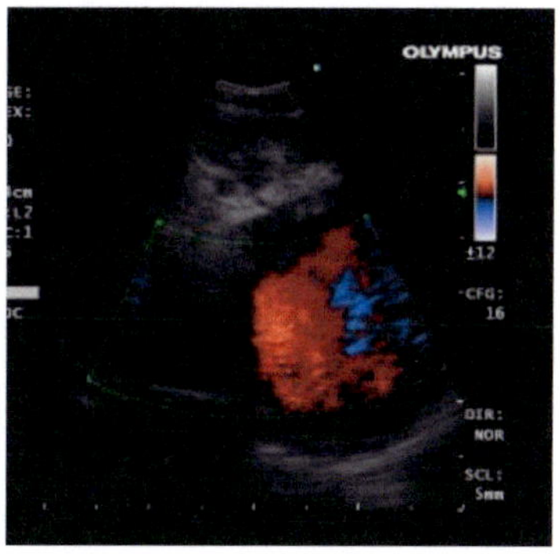

REFERENCES:

1. Murgu S and Colt HG. Practical approach to planning endobronchial ultrasound-guided transbronchial needle aspiration of left lower paratracheal lymph node (level 4L). Egyptian J Bronch 2009;3(2):169-171.
2. Colt HG, Davoudi M, Murgu SD. Scientific evidence and principles for the use of endobronchial ultrasound and EBUS-TBNA. Expert Rev Med Dev. 2011;8:493-513.

Question I.18: Which of the following ultrasound parameters is determined by the transducer's frequency?

A. Image resolution

B. Depth of penetration

C. Attenuation

D. All of the above

Answer I.18: D.

Frequency represents a specific number of vibration cycles per second, measured in units of hertz. EBUS frequencies range from of 5 to 30 MHz. Dedicated EBUS-TBNA bronchoscopes allow a change in frequency from 5 to12 MHz, while available high frequency EBUS systems use frequencies of 20 to 30 MHz[1]. Resolution refers to a system's capacity to distinguish small objects from others, determined by the frequency and duration of the transmitted sound wave. Axial resolution represents the ability to resolve objects within the imaging plane at different depths, and depends on US pulse duration which depends on frequency. The higher the frequency, the higher the resolution and vice versa. Penetration refers to the distance between an imaged area and the transducer. Maximum penetration depth depends on frequency, but this relationship is indirect (see Figure below). Higher frequencies (20 MHz) do not penetrate as deep as lower ones (7.5 MHz). Superficial structures are thus better visualized using higher frequencies, while deeper structures are better visualized using lower frequency transducers. 20 MHz EBUS radial probes are used for imaging airway wall layers, while 7.5 MHz EBUS probes are used for deeper structures such as lymph nodes and blood vessels (see Figure below). In

Figure A, the radial probe (20 MHz) inside a subglottic stenosis at the level of the cricoid cartilage shows the hypertrophic stenotic tissue and the intact cricoid cartilage, but the deeper structures are not visualized. In Figure B, the curved linear EBUS transducer (7.5 MHz) faces the right antero-lateral wall of the lower trachea and the corresponding EBUS image shows the right lower paratracheal lymph node, the superior vena cava and the distal normal lung parenchyma but details of the airway wall structures could not be assessed. Attenuation is loss of energy caused by absorption (vibration of the US wave is converted by friction into heat). Attenuation depends on the medium and frequency, being higher in air than in water and increasing with higher frequencies.

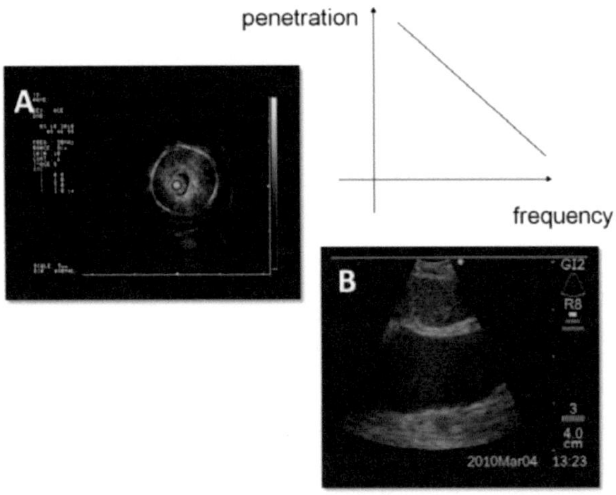

REFERENCES:

1. Colt HG, Davoudi M, Murgu SD. Scientific evidence and principles for the use of endobronchial ultrasound and EBUS-TBNA. Expert Review of Medical Devices. 2010 (in press).

Question I.19: Which of the following processes does not degrade ultrasound image quality while ultrasound waves penetrate through tissues?

A. Reflection

B. Refraction

C. Scattering

D. Attenuation

Answer I.19: A.

When the ultrasound beam strikes an interface, it undergoes refraction, scattering, and attenuation, all of which lead to image quality degradation while imaging deeper tissue structures. Refraction represents a change in direction of the incident US beam. Scattering is the spread of the US beam in different directions. Reflected waves are not transmitted in a tissue, but they bounce back similar to light reflecting off a mirror (see Figure below).

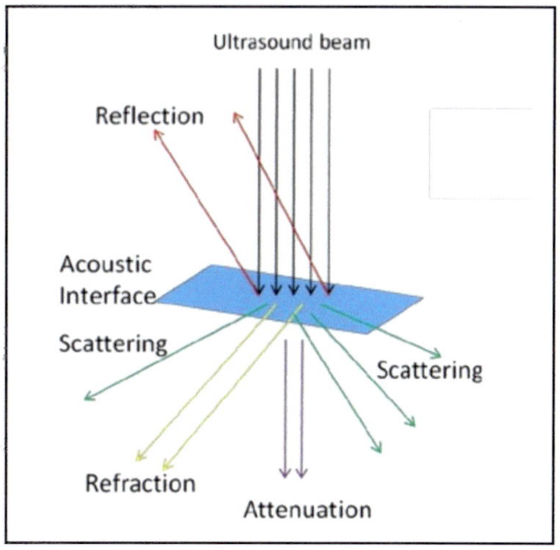

Question I.20: While performing EBUS examination of the mediastinum you obtain the image shown below. To increase the brightness of the entire image you tell your assistant to:

A. Increase the gain

B. Increase the depth

C. Switch to Doppler mode

D. There is nothing you can do

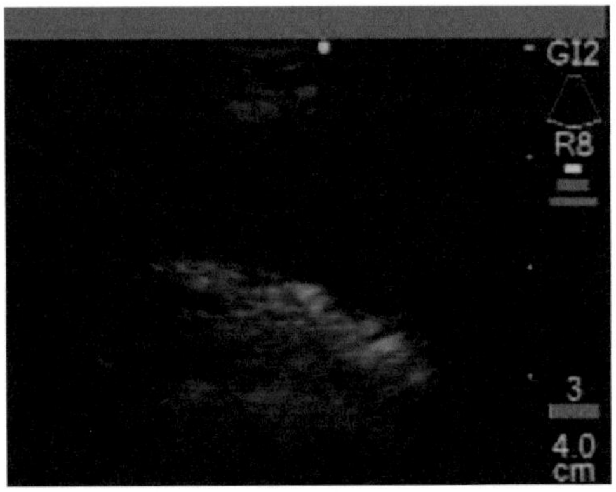

Answer I.20: A.

This image is displayed at low gain. Gain represents the function for adjusting the brightness of the image in its entirety. Changing gain makes the image brighter or darker but differences in brightness between light and dark areas are unchanged (see Figure below). Contrast, on the other hand, adjusts the brightness difference between light and dark areas of the image by varying signal strength and is particularly useful for echo-poor structures. Doppler mode is useful for distinguishing vessels from other structures, but switching to Doppler mode does not improve the image quality.

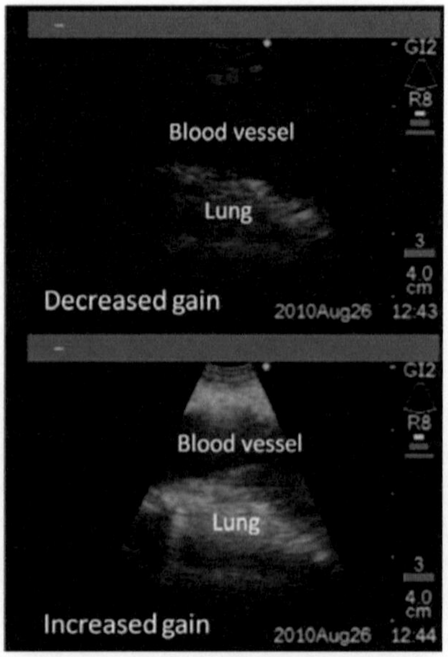

Question I.21: An asymptomatic 72 year-old woman, a 15 pack year former smoker with a remote history of breast cancer, is referred to you after a CT scan of the chest revealed a 2 cm subcarinal lymph node. In your conversation with the patient, you inform her that from among the possible causes of her enlarged node, EBUS-TBNA is least effective to diagnose:

A. Primary lung cancer

B. Recurrent breast cancer

C. Sarcoidosis

D. Lymphoma

Answer I.21: D.

All of the disorders listed above can be diagnosed by EBUS-TBNA. Meta-analysis shows that EBUS-TBNA has an overall pooled sensitivity of 93% and specificity of 100% with the highest pooled sensitivity of 97% was seen in studies that included on-site cytology[1]. The sensitivity and specificity of EBUS-TBNA for diagnosis of mediastinal and hilar lymph node metastasis from non-pulmonary tumors have been reported to be as high as 92.0% and 100%, respectively. The tumors encountered included colorectal, head and neck, ovarian, breast, esophageal, hepatocellular, prostate, renal, and germ cell cancers and malignant melanoma[2]. For sarcoidosis, EBUS-TBNA has a sensitivity and specificity of 83.3% and 100% respectively[3]. In a high pre-test probability population, the sensitivity may be even higher than 90% [4]. For lymphoma, a study evaluating patients with high pre-test probability for lymphoma in a tertiary cancer center revealed an overall sensitivity was 90.9% and specificity of 100% [5]. Larger, prospective studies showed that the sensitivity and specificity of EBUS-TBNA for definitive diagnosis of lymphoma were 57% and 100%, respectively[6]. While the diagnostic accuracy of EBUS-TBNA for lymphoma is lower than that for other cancers, the procedure appears to be appropriate for patients with isolated mediastinal lymphadenopathy, considering the low incidence of lymphoma in this population and the significant proportion of such patients (76%) in whom surgical biopsy might be avoided[6].

REFERENCES:

1. Gu P, Zhao Y, Jiang L, Zhang W, Xin Y, Han B. Endobronchial ultrasound-guided transbronchial needle aspiration for staging of lung cancer: A systematic review and meta-analysis. Eur J Cancer. 45, 1389-1396 (2009).
2. Nakajima T, Yasufuku K, Iyoda A, et al. The evaluation of lymph node metastasis by endobronchial ultrasound-guided transbronchial needle aspiration: Crucial for selection of surgical candidates with metastatic lung tumors. J Thorac Cardiovasc Surg. 134, 1485-1490 (2007).
3. Tremblay A, Stather DR, MacEachern P, Khalil M, Field SK. A Randomized Controlled Trial of Standard vs Endobronchial Ultrasonography-Guided Transbronchial Needle Aspiration in Patients With Suspected Sarcoidosis. Chest. 136, 340-346 (2009).
4. Wong M, Yasufuku K, Nakajima T, et al. Endobronchial ultrasound: new insight for the diagnosis of sarcoidosis. Eur Respir J. 29(6), 1182-1186 (2007).

5. Kennedy MP, Jimenez CA, Bruzzi Jf, et al. Endobronchial ultrasound-guided transbronchial needle aspiration in the diagnosis of lymphoma. Thorax. 63, 360-365 (2008).
6. Steinfort DP, Conron M, Tsui A, et al. Endobronchial ultrasound-guided transbronchial needle aspiration for the evaluation of suspected lymphoma. J Thorac Oncol. 5(6), 8 04-809 (2010).

Question I.22: High frequency endobronchial ultrasonography has been successfully used for which of the following applications:

A. Determining the depth of tumor invasion inside the airway wall.
B. Screening patient with airway early lung cancer who could be cured by PDT.
C. Detecting cartilage abnormalities in various forms of malacia.
D. All of the above.

Answer I.22: D.

Several investigators showed the utility of high frequency EBUS using 20 MHz radial probe in determining the depth of tumor invasion in centrally located lung cancer. This is possible because EBUS can reveal the laminar structure of the airway wall[1, 2]. Lesions which have not invaded the cartilage layer may be treated surgically, or for inoperable patients, using intraluminal modalities such as brachytherapy, laser ablation or photodynamic therapy (PDT). Studies of patients with central airway early lung cancer diagnosed as intracartilaginous by EBUS and subsequently treated by PDT show high long-term complete remission rates[3, 4]. There are many reports of potential roles for EBUS in the diagnosis of benign airway wall disorders such as asthma, malacia due to relapsing polychondritis, tuberculosis, extrinsic compression from vascular structures, chronic tracheatis and excessive dynamic airway collapse.

REFERENCES:

1. Kurimoto N, Murayama M, Yoshioka S, Nishisaka T, Inai K, Dohi K. Assessment of Usefulness of Endobronchial Ultrasonography in Determination of Depth of Tracheobronchial Tumor Invasion. Chest. 115, 1500-1506 (1999).
2. Baba M, Sekine Y, Suzuki M et al. Correlation between endobronchial ultrasonography (EBUS) images and histologic findings in normal and tumor-invaded bronchial wall. Lung Cancer. 35, 65-71 (2002).
3. Miyazu Y, Miyazawa T, Kurimoto N, IwamotoY, Kanoh K, Kohno N. Endobronchial Ultrasonography in the Assessment of Centrally Located Early-Stage Lung Cancer before Photodynamic Therapy. Am J Respir Crit Care Med. 165, 832-837(2002).
4. Takahashi H, Sagawa M, Sato M, et al. A prospective evaluation of transbronchial ultrasonography for assessment of depth of invasion in early bronchogenic squamous cell carcinoma. Lung Cancer. 42, 43-49 (2003).

Question I.23: Which of the following anesthesia methods would you employ to perform EBUS-TBNA for a patient with the lymph node shown belo\

A. General anesthesia with endotracheal intubation.

B. General anesthesia with laryngeal mask airway.

C. Moderate sedation.

D. Local laryngotracheal analgesia.

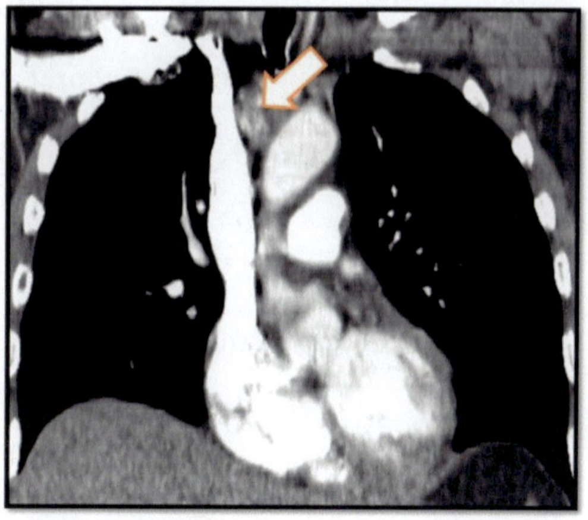

Answer I.23: B.

This coronal CT scan view shows the right upper paratracheal (station 2R) lymph node station. Station 2R includes nodes extending to the left lateral border of the trachea. The upper border is the apex of the right lung and pleural space, and in the midline, the upper border of the manubrium while the lower border is the intersection of caudal margin of innominate vein with the trachea. Laryngeal mask airway (LMA) permits evaluation of the upper paratracheal nodes (namely 2R and 2L) which may not be accessible if an endotracheal tube (ETT) is used[1]. This is because these nodes are located adjacent to a region of the trachea that is covered by the endotracheal tube, even if the cuff is inflated immediately below the vocal cords. It is probably preferable to sample these regions by passing the scope passed directly through an LMA or an oral biteblock[2]. EBUS can be performed under moderate sedation in the bronchoscopy suite. This may potentially result in greater safety and cost savings compared to general anesthesia, but visualization and biopsy of smaller nodes is technically more difficult than with general anesthesia[3]. Most published studies of EBUS-TBNA showing high diagnostic yields were in fact performed under general anesthesia. Long bronchoscopic procedures can be uncomfortable for patients and it may be difficult to keep patients from coughing or otherwise moving without general anesthesia. Many experts feel that EBUS-TNBA (using the EBUS scope with an outer diameter of 6.7 mm and requiring placement of the scope in the high trachea for sampling station 2R), is unlikely to be done well and comfortably (for the patient as well as the bronchoscopist) without good anesthesia.

REFERENCES:

1. Douadi Y, Bentayeb H, Malinowski S et al. Anaesthesia for bronchial echoendoscopy: experience with the laryngeal mask. Rev Mal Respir. 2010; 27 :37-41
2. Sarkiss M, Kennedy M, Riedel B et al. Anesthesia technique for endobronchial ultrasound-guided fine needle aspiration of mediastinal lymph node. J Cardiothorac Vasc Anesth 2007; 21:892–896
3. Kennedy MP, Shweihat Y, Sarkiss M, Eapen GA. Complete mediastinal and hilar lymph node staging of primary lung cancer by endobronchial ultrasound: moderate sedation or general anesthesia? Chest 2008; 134; 1350-1351

Question I.24: While performing EBUS-TBNA, after the needle system is secured on the scope your next step should be:

A. Release the needle screw

B. Release the sheath screw

C. Agitate the stylet several times in and out of the needle-sheath

D. Advance the sheath until it touches the airway wall

Answer 24: B.

Once the target node is selected, EBUS-TBNA can be performed as summarized in the table. Once the needle is secured on the scope (Step 2), the sheath screw is released (Step 3) by twisting the inferior screw (see Figure below).

Step Number	Description
Step 1	The biopsy needle is passed through the biopsy channel.
Step 2	The housing is secured to the bronchoscope by a flange.
Step 3	The sheath is released by twisting the inferior screw.
Step 4	With the node visualized by US, the sheath is advanced out of the end of the scope until it slightly touches the airway wall. It is therefore safe to advance the needle.
Step 5	The needle screw, located superiorly, is then released.
Step 6	The needle is advanced into the lymph node using a quick jab. During this process the needle may push the airway wall away from the balloon. Thus the transducer –wall interface is lost and the image may show reverberation artifacts. The problem is overcome by gently advancing the scope and /or further inflating the balloon.
Step 7	Visualize needle entering target node
Step 8	Move the stylet in and out a few times to dislodge bronchial wall debris.
Step 9	Remove the stylet
Step 10	The syringe is applied to the biopsy needle.
Step 11	Suction is applied at usually negative 20 ml of air.
Step 12	Pass the needle in and out of the node 15 times
Step 13	Suction is then released.
Step 14	Retract the needle into the sheath
Step 15	The needle housing is unlocked and the needle and the sheath are removed together and the aspirated material is smeared onto glass slides.

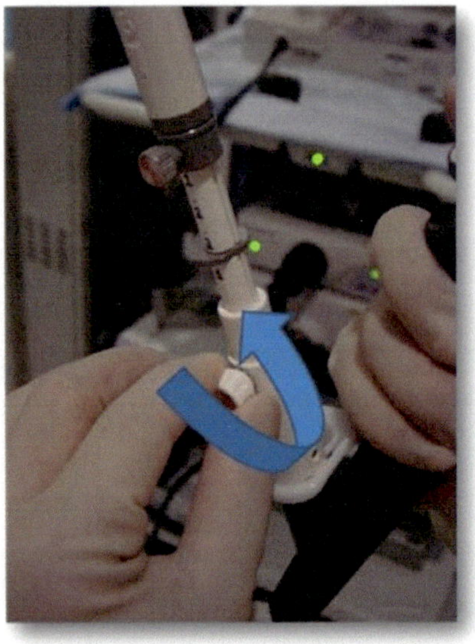

REFERENCES:

1. S Murgu, M Davoudi, H Colt. EBUS Step by Step video available on YouTube (BronchOrg channel) 9/10/10.

Question I.25: While performing EBUS-TBNA, once the needle is visualized inside the node, the next thing you do is to:

A. Remove the stylet and attach the syringe

B. Move the stylet in and out a few times

C. Pass the needle in and out 10-15 times

D. Apply suction with approximately negative 20 ml of air

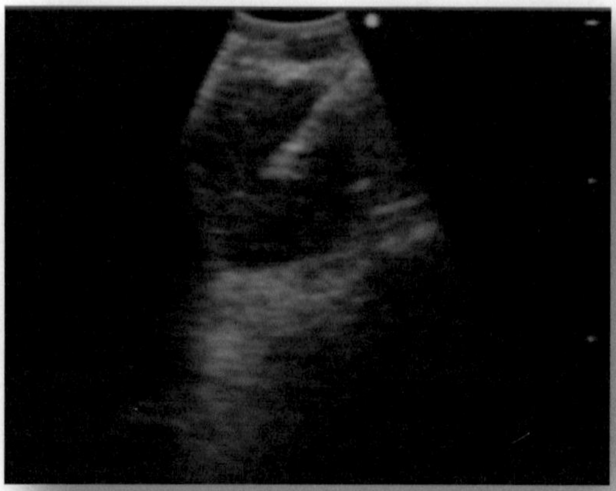

Answer I.25: B.

Once the needle is visualized within the lymph node, the stylet is moved in an out a few times to dislodge any bronchial epithelium that may have entered the needle (Figure A) and only afterwards the stylet is removed (Figure B), the syringe is attached (Figure C) and suction is applied (Figure D). Only afterwards the needle is passed in and out 10- 15 times during aspiration.

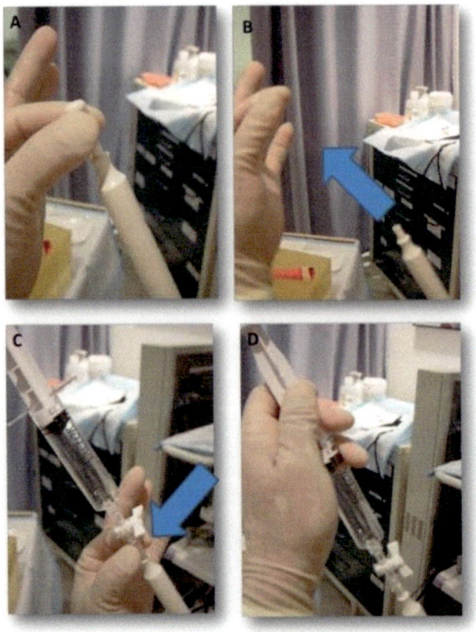

Question I.26: While performing EBUS-TBNA, after the second aspirate your cytopathologist colleague tells you that there are only benign bronchial cells seen on a Diff-Quick stain. Your answer should be:

A. "It's impossible! I clearly see the needle inside the node."
B. "I don't get it! You should either see lymphocytes or malignant cells."
C. "OK! That is all I can do. I will stop the procedure"
D. "OK! That is not unusual. I will proceed with more aspirates"

Answer I.26: D.

Understanding what is actually occurring inside the lymph node will help avoid frustration when aspiration results are not quite what one might expect (for example when bronchial cells are seen, or blood is aspirated even though you are certain you are in the node). In this example, bronchial wall debris is pushed inside the node when the stylet is moved back and forth. Not uncommonly, the material initially dislodged is aspirated back in the syringe once suction is applied (see Figure below). Images A, B, C and D are consecutive images captured from a video showing EBUS-TBNA during the aspiration process. In A, the stylet pushed the bronchial wall debris inside the node. In B, the needle is retracted and the debris becomes evidently dislodged from the needle. In C, the needle is advanced during the 10-15 revolutions while aspiration is in process. In D, the debris had completely disappeared, being aspirated in the syringe. The right decision, therefore, is to proceed with additional sampling despite the initially unsatisfactory result.

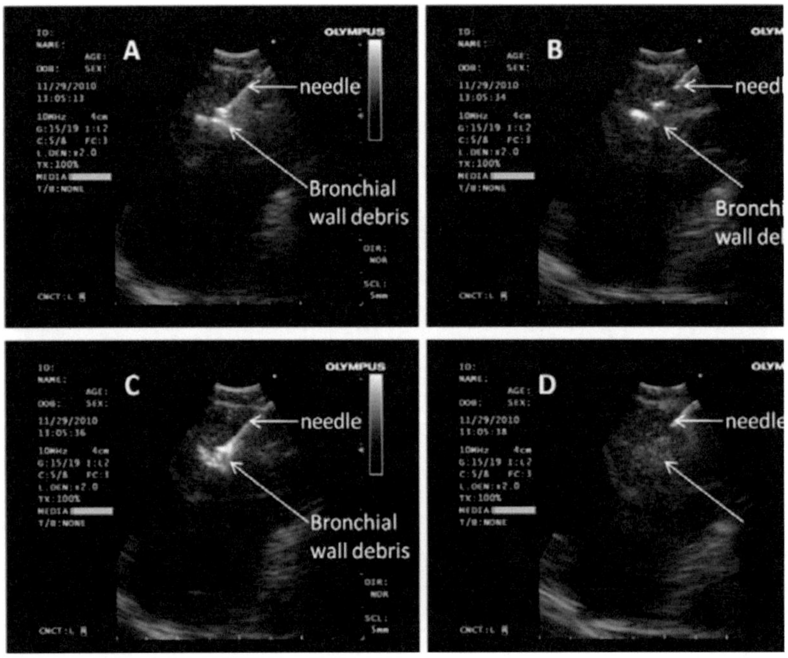

Question I.27: While performing EBUS imaging of the mediastinal structures you placed your bronchoscope just proximal to the main carina and pointed the transducer anteriorly (A). The structure shown at 12 o'clock position on the display monitor (B) represents the:

A. Lymph node station 10 R

B. Lymph node station 3a

C. Lymph node station 5

D. Lymph node station 4R

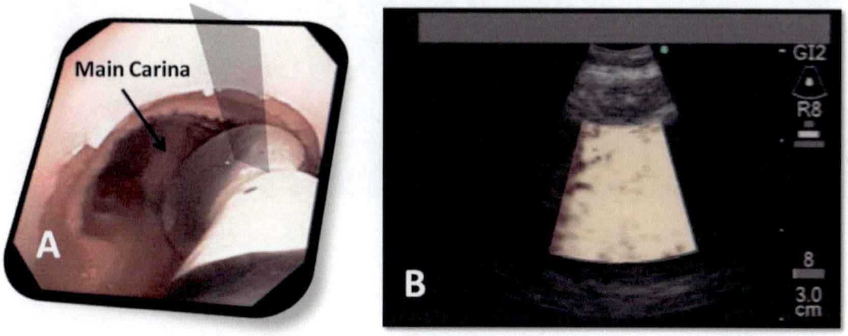

Answer I.27: D.

Station 4R includes right lower paratracheal nodes, and pretracheal nodes extending to the left lateral border of trachea. Therefore, when the scope is pointed anteriorly at the level of main carina, the node seen is still the right lower paratracheal (station 4R). The Doppler positive vessel behind it represents the ascending aorta (see Figure below). Station 10 R includes nodes immediately adjacent to the main bronchus and hilar vessels including the proximal portions of the pulmonary veins and main pulmonary artery with the upper border, the lower rim of the azygos vein on the right and the lower border, the interlobar region between right upper lobe and bronchus intermedius. Station 5 (aorto-pulmonary window), is to the left of the trachea and not adjacent to the airway. Station 3a (prevascular) is in the anterior mediastinum and not adjacent to the airway. Its border on the right is the upper border of the apex of the chest, its lower border is at the level of the carina and its anterior border is the posterior aspect of sternum while its posterior border is the anterior border of superior vena cava.

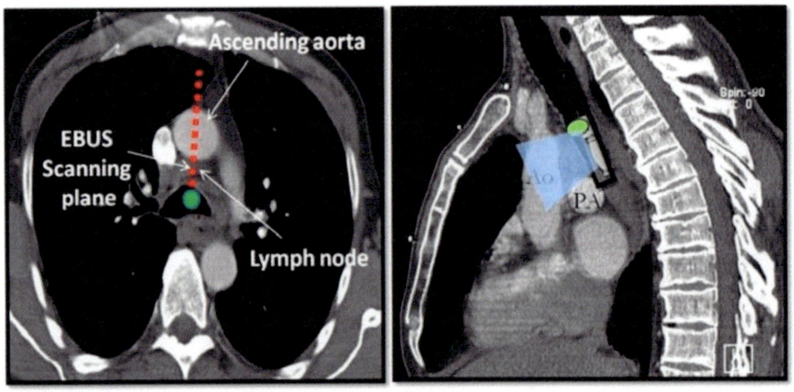

Question I.28: With the EBUS scope in the proximal bronchus intermedius and with the transducer pointed towards the right lateral wall, the following image is displayed on the monitor. The marked structure (arrow) represents:

A. Lymph node station 10R

B. Lymph node station 11R superior

C. Lymph node station 11R inferior

D. Interlobar artery

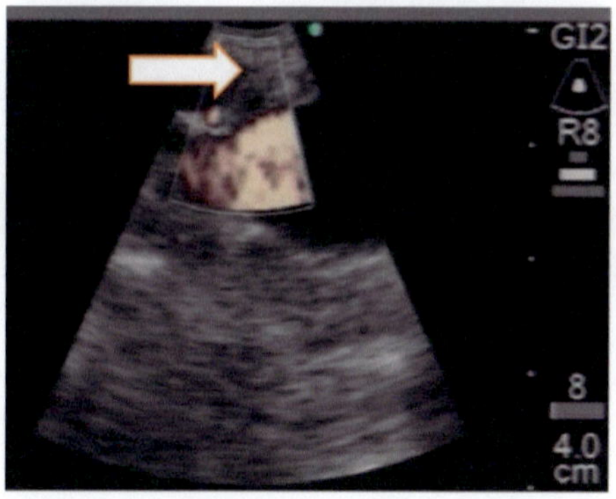

Answer I.28: B.

With the scope at that location and orientation (see Figure below), the visualized lymph node pointed to in the image is the right superior interlobar node (station 11R s). Station 11R superior is comprised of the nodes between the right upper lobe bronchus and bronchus intermedius. Station 11R inferior is between the middle and the right lower lobe bronchi and is visualized with the scope positioned in the proximal right lower lobe and the transducer pointed towards the right lateral wall. Station 10 R includes nodes immediately adjacent to the right main bronchus and hilar vessels including the proximal portions of the pulmonary veins and main pulmonary artery. This station is visualized by gently advancing the scope from the carina down on the RMB, with the transducer pointed antero-laterally towards 2-o'clock position (orientation based on patient being scoped from the head). The interlobar artery is the anechoic Doppler positive structure adjacent to the node (see Figure below).

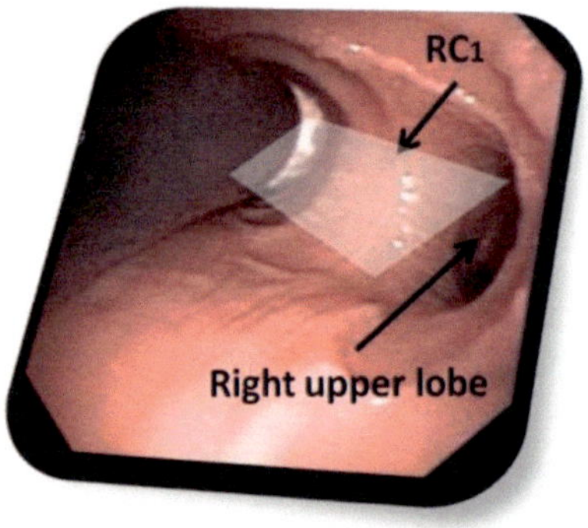

Question I.29: A patient with a right upper lobe mass underwent an integrated PET-CT which showed a PET positive level 11R and PET negative level 7 lymph nodes. After white light bronchoscopy revealed no endobronchial abnormalities, you proceed with EBUS for diagnosis and staging. The first thing you should do is to:

A. Sample station 7 since the diagnostic yield is higher than from station 11R

B. Sample station 11R since it's PET positive

C. Evaluate and sample left sided mediastinal lymph nodes, if present

D. Evaluate and sample any pre-carinal lymph nodes, if present

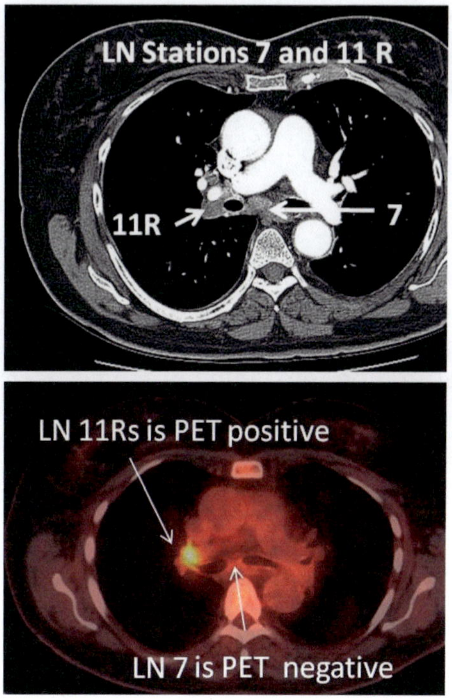

Answer I.29: C.

Overall, the TBNA diagnostic yield is higher from subcarinal nodes than from other stations. This holds true both for conventional and for EBUS-TBNA. This would argue for initially sampling the subcarinal node. However, selecting the PET positive node for TBNA could increase the sensitivity of the procedure. Data from a meta-analysis showed that the subgroup of patients who were selected on the basis of CT or PET positive results had higher pooled sensitivity (0.94, 95% CI 0.93–0.96) than the subgroup of patients without any selection of CT or PET (0.76, 95% CI 0.65–0.85) ($p < 0.05$)[1]. When performed for diagnosis and staging purposes, however, EBUS-TBNA should be performed first from N3 nodes, followed by N2 nodes and for diagnosis, when necessary, N1 nodes. If N3 nodes were found to be positive for malignancy on rapid on-site cytological evaluation, the procedure could be terminated. In this case N3 nodes are the contralateral (left) sided mediastinal nodes. The pre-carinal nodes are part of station 4R, thus in this case, are still N2 nodes.

REFERENCES:

1. Gu P, Zhao Y, Jiang L, Zhang W, Xin Y, Han B. Endobronchial ultrasound-guided transbronchial needle aspiration for staging of lung cancer: A systematic review and meta-analysis. Eur J Cancer. 45, 1389-1396 (2009).

Question I.30: While performing EBUS-TBNA from a right lower paratracheal node in an asymptomatic 30 year old non-smoking African American woman, the cytologist tells you that there is "non-caseating granulomatous inflammation". Based on this information, which of the following is the most likely diagnosis?

A. Primary lung carcinoma
B. Sarcoidosis
C. Tuberculosis
D. Lymphoma

Answer I.30: B.

This patient has a high pre-test probability for sarcoidosis. In sarcoidosis, lymph node enlargement is usually seen in the right paratracheal, aorto-pulmonary window and hilar regions. EBUS-TBNA cytology specimens when used in conjunction with clinical findings, radiological and laboratory investigations, is a useful tool in the diagnosis of sarcoidosis. Demonstration of granulomas remains an essential criterion, but as granulomatous inflammation can be seen in host of conditions, it is necessary to exclude all possible causes, as well as to correlate with other findings, before arriving at the diagnosis of sarcoidosis. One should keep in mind that lymph nodes harboring both necrotizing and non-necrotizing granulomas and malignancy have been described[1, 2]. In general, to establish a diagnosis of sarcoidosis it is necessary that granulomata must be present in two or more organs, with no agent known to cause a granulomatous response being identified. A search should be made for other causes of granulomatous inflammation, including mycobacteria, fungi, parasites, and foreign bodies. Tuberculosis may also present as non-caseating, and if suspected, the specimen should be also sent for culture. One major pitfall may be finding non-caseating granulomas in sarcoid reaction. These are morphologically identical to the granulomas of sarcoidosis. Sarcoid reactions have been reported in patients with various lymphomas, non-small cell carcinoma of the lung, and germ cell neoplasm, either in lymph nodes draining the malignancy or in remote lymph node stations[3]. These sarcoid-like granulomas appear to represent a local T cell-mediated immune reaction. The diagnosis of lymphoma may be more controversial, although the use of flow cytometry, molecular biology techniques and immunohistochemistry on cell block preps may provide enough information for a definitive diagnosis or robust data for a diagnosis of lymphoma without any further specification.

REFERENCES:

1. Pandey M, Abraham EK, Chandramohan K, et al. Tuberculosis and metastatic carcinoma coexistence in axillary lymph node: a case report. World J Surg Oncol. 2003;1:3.
2. Laurberg P. Sarcoid reactions in pulmonary neoplasms. Scand J Respir Dis. 1975; 56:20-27.
3. Steinfort DP, Irving LB. Sarcoidal reactions in regional lymph nodes of patients with non-small cell lung cancer: Incidence and implications for minimally invasive staging with endobronchial ultrasound. Lung Cancer 2009;66:305–308.

The Essential EBUS Bronchoscopist©

MODULE 1 Post-test

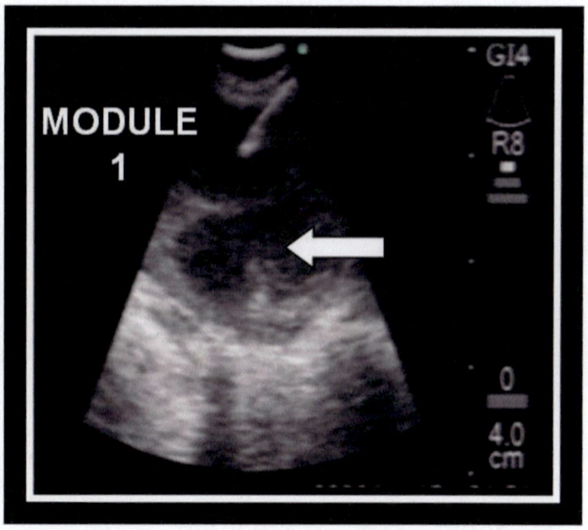

You have now completed studying this component of the Essential EBUS Bronchoscopist©.

You should now take the post-test. All post-tests are multiple-choice, single BEST answer. Please remember that while many programs consider 70% correct responses a passing grade, the learner's "target" score should be 100%.

Please send us your comments regarding your participation in this international educational endeavor
by contacting your national bronchology association, or by emailing us at www.bronchoscopy.org.

The Essential EBUS Bronchoscopist
Post test

Please answer the following TEN multiple choice questions. There is a "single" best answer for each question. Your target score is 100% correct responses, although many institutions will use 70% correct responses as a satisfactory grade.

Question 1. EBUS TBNA and conventional TBNA are of equal efficacy for sampling which of the following nodal stations?

A. Station 10R
B. Station 4L
C. Station 7
D. Station 5

Question 2. Maximum penetration depth of an ultrasound wave depends most on:

A. Frequency
B. Resolution
C. Tissue color
D. Pulse duration

Question 3. Representative cytology specimens are best obtained by:

A. Aspirating from the center of the lymph node
B. Noting more than 10% cellularity composed of lymphocytes
C. Repeated aspiration attempts until a tissue core is obtained
D. Aspirating from the periphery of the lymph node

Question 4. When the water-filled balloon is not in contact with the airway wall, which of the following artefacts is usually seen?

A. Tadpole tail artefact
B. Comet tail artefact
C. Reverberation artefact
D. Acoustic shadowing

Question 5. The typical coagulation necrosis sign seen during EBUS includes which of the following?

A. Hyperechoic area with blood flow
B. Hypoechoic area with blood flow
C. Hypoechoic area without blood flow that sometimes occupies the entire node
D. Hypoechoic area without blood flow, usually in a small section of the node

Question 6. In a patient with left upper lobe adenocarcinoma requiring mediastinal staging, which of the following nodal stations should be sampled first?

A. The enlarged, but PET negative contralateral lower paratracheal node
B. The enlarged but PET negative subcarinal node
C. The enlarged ipsilateral PET positive hilar node
D. The enlarged ipsilateral PET positive lower paratracheal node

Question 7. Which of the following is an attenuation artefact?

A. The acoustic shadow sign
B. The comet tail sign
C. The pleural reflection sign
D. The hepatization lung sign

Question 8. Which of the following is true about lower frequency ultrasound such as that used in EBUS convex probe procedures?

A. Penetration depth is greater than with higher frequency probes
B. Superficial structures are better visualized than with higher frequency probes
C. Airway wall layers are better visualized than with higher frequency probes
D. Resolution is higher than with higher frequency probes

Question 9. Laryngeal mask airways (LMA) are helpful while performing EBUS – TBNA because:

A. LMAs can be placed without use of a general anesthetic or hypnotic agent
B. LMAs have a minimal risk of aspiration compared to performing EBUS without an indwelling airway.
C. LMAs facilitate access to level 2 lymph nodes compared to endotracheal tubes.
D. LMAs allow faster awakening compared to performing EBUS with an endotracheal tube.

Question 10. Which of the following EBUS-TBNA related complications has the greatest impact on patient management?

A. Inability to sample a level 7 node because of scope breakage during the procedure
B. False negative sampling of a contralateral paratracheal node
C. False negative sampling of an ipsilateral level 10 node
D. Inability to penetrate through the lymph node capsule

NOTES

The EBUS Bronchoscopist©

Answers to post-tests

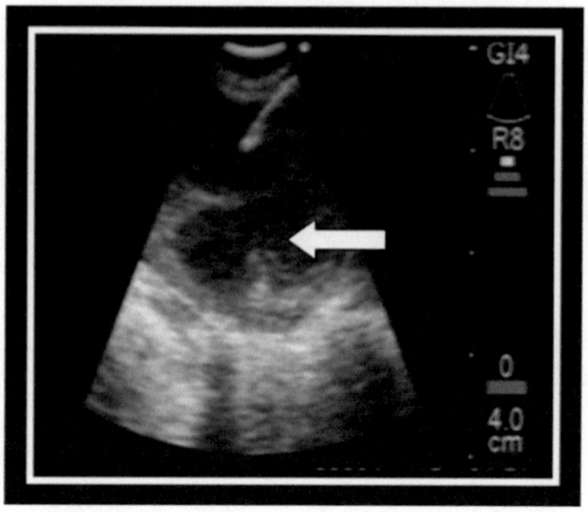

Post-tests are multiple choice, single BEST answer.

While many programs consider 70% correct responses a passing grade, the learner's "target" score should be 100%.

EBUS Bronchoscopist© Post-test Answers

Module 1

1. C
2. A
3. D
4. C
5. C
6. A
7. A
8. A
9. C
10. B

CONGRATULATIONS

You have now completed

The Essential EBUS Bronchoscopist

This is an important achievement on your journey to competency. We know that you will use what you have learned to enhance your bronchoscopy skills.

This reading assignment is complementary to other components of the Endobronchial Ultrasound and EBUS-guided TBNA curriculum, just one part in your quest to become a more competent and knowledgeable bronchoscopist.

We encourage you to attend national and international professional medical society meetings around the world so that you may share your experiences with your colleagues. We also urge you to explore the Bronchoscopy International website (www.Bronchoscopy.org) for other learning materials, and to search instructional videos on the BronchOrg YouTube site. (See Video)

We look forward to receiving your comments regarding this and other components of The Bronchoscopy Education Project.

Please do not hesitate to contact your regional bronchology association, or email us at www.bronchoscopy.org

Thank you for participating in The Bronchoscopy Education Project!

§

About the Authors

Henri Colt MD is an internationally recognized physician leader, professor emeritus of medicine, teacher, award-winning educator, and ethicist. In addition to his academic achievements, leadership positions in professional medical societies, and hundreds of lectures in more than ninety countries, he has published numerous articles and book chapters on all aspects of interventional pulmonology. His work on competency-oriented processes and procedures pertaining to bronchoscopy education is being emulated by physician leaders around the globe.

In founding Bronchoscopy International, Henri surrounds himself with like-minded individuals dedicated to serving populations in need, and to changing the paradigm of medical education so that patients need no longer suffer the burden of procedure-related learning. When he is not teaching, you may find him enjoying desert trails or sunny beaches in Southern California.

Septimiu Murgu MD is a chest physician whose primary clinical and research interests include the diagnosis and management of lung cancer, and the pathophysiology, airway dynamics and management of expiratory central airway collapse. A physicist at heart, Dr. Murgu has an insatiable curiosity that prompts him to explore ways that acoustic and optical technologies might assist in the study of airway disorders.

He is the coauthor of the textbook *The Patient-Centered Approach to Central Airways Disorders*, as well as of numerous original research papers and review articles. A devoted teacher, Tim participates in numerous training courses and faculty development programs organized in collaboration with Bronchoscopy International as well as national and international professional medical organizations.

Made in the USA
Monee, IL
19 June 2026

54848123R00050